Introduction to Urological Nursing

Introduction to Urological Nursing

Edited by

PHILIP DOWNEY BSc(HONS), RGN
The Royal Liverpool Hospitals NHS Trust

W

WHURR PUBLISHERS
LONDON AND PHILADELPHIA

© 2000 Whurr Publishers Ltd
First published 2000 by
Whurr Publishers Ltd
19b Compton Terrace, London N1 2UN, England and
325 Chestnut Street, Philadelphia PA 19106, USA.

Reprinted 2001

British Library Cataloguing in Publication Data
A catalogue record for this book is available from the British
Library.

ISBN 1 86156 150 4

Printed and bound in the UK by Athenæum Press Ltd,
Gateshead, Tyne & Wear

Contents

Contributors

Caroline BARROW BSc(Hons), RSCN
Urology Nurse Specialist, Royal Liverpool Childrens Hospital (Alder Hey), Liverpool

Jeanne BECKETT BSc(Hons), RGN, SCM, DipN
Senior Staff Nurse (Urology), Glan Clwyd Hospital, Boddelwyddn, North Wales

Gaynor BOND DipHE, RN
Staff Nurse (Urology), The Royal Liverpool University Hospitals NHS Trust, Liverpool

David BURNS BSc(Hons), CertEd, RGN, RNT
Teacher, Edge Hill University College, Ormskirk, Lancashire

Philip DOWNEY BSc(Hons) RGN
Ward Manager (Urology), The Royal Liverpool University Hospitals NHS Trust, Liverpool

Lisa GRANT DipHE, RN
Staff Nurse (Urology), The Royal Liverpool University Hospitals NHS Trust, Liverpool

Andrea GRIFFIN BN(Hons), RN, ONC
Staff Nurse (General Surgery), Manchester Royal Infirmary, Manchester

Janet HALL RGN, DPSN
Ward Manager (Urology), Glan Clwyd Hospital, Boddelwyddn, North Wales

David LYNES BSc(Hons), EN(G), RGN, RNT, DPSN
National Training Manager, Respiratory Education Resource Centre, University Hospital Aintree, Liverpool

Ian PEATE BED(Hons), MA(Lond), EN(G), RGN, DipN(Lond), RNT
Senior Lecturer, University of Hertfordshire, Hertfordshire
Penny WESTBROOK BN(Hons), RN, DNC
Staff Nurse (Medicine), West Cumberland Hospital, Whitehaven, Cumbria

Preface

Change is inevitable, and to be expected. With changes in nursing care comes advancement and an altering of priorities. Urology as a speciality is constantly changing and advancing, and this is reflected in the responsibilities of nurses working within the speciality. The practising nurse requires a textbook to support him or her through their time in urology.

This book provides a comprehensive, up-to-date guide to urology, giving information on all aspects of the genitourinary system. There is a chapter covering the detailed anatomy and physiology to allow nurses to gain an insight into the normal functions of the organs involved, and therefore an understanding of the treatments available.

The text is aimed at the nurse about to qualify, and also nurses currently specializing in urology, who want an easy-to-read textbook for reference in their work. It is a valuable source of information, providing the latest and most up-to-date material to help the practising nurse well into the 21st Century.

Philip Downey

Acknowledgements

I would like to thank my wife, Kim, for all her help, encouragement and support during the writing of this book.

I would also like to thank my manager, John James (Directorate Manager, The Royal Liverpool University Hospitals Trust), for his advice and suggestions. His encouragement and empathy were very much appreciated.

Finally, I would like to thank the authors of the chapters. Without them and their enthusiasm, this book would never have been written.

Philip Downey

Abbreviations

AFB	Acid fast bacillus
BCG	Calmette–Guérin bacillus
BPH	Benign prostatic hyperplasia
CAL	Computer-assisted learning
CAPD	Continuous (or chronic) ambulatory peritoneal dialysis
CISC	Clean intermittent self-catheterization
CT	Computerized tomography
CUDS	Closed urinary drainage system
DoH	Department of Health
DRE	Digital rectal examination
DVU	Direct visual urethrotomy
ECG	Electrocardiogram
ESRF	End stage renal failure
FSH	Follicle-stimulating hormone
GFR	Glomerular filtration rate
GP	General (medical) practitioner
IV	Intravenous
IVU	Intravenous urography
KUB	Kidney, ureter and bladder X-ray
LH	Luteinizing hormone
MCU	Micturating cystourethrogram
MRI	Magnetic resonance imaging
MUSE	Medicated urethral system for erection
PCA	Patient-controlled analgesia
PSA	Prostate-specific antigen
PUV	Posterior urethral valves
PVC	Polyvinyl chloride

T3   Trans wave thermotherapy
TB   Tuberculosis bacillus
TSE   Testicular self-examination
TUIP   Transurethral incision of prostate
TUNA   Transurethral needle abliteration
TURBT   Transurethral resection of bladder tumour
TURP   Transurethral resection of prostate
TURT   Transurethral resection of tumour (bladder)
UKCC   United Kingdom Central Council for Nursing, Midwifery
            and Health Visiting

Introduction

An Introduction to Urological Nursing is a largely clinically based book providing the latest information concerned with the delivery of holistic nursing care. It is written by nurses for nurses, and is aimed at both the student nurse about to qualify and the nurse currently practising in the speciality.

Nurses in both categories require an easy-to-read textbook giving them an adequate amount of detail to aid them in their practice. All nurses in the clinical setting are aware of time constraints within their work schedule. As a result, information needs to be readily available, accessible, quick to find and written in a simple and straightforward manner. This book is written in this style.

It is wise to start with the basics, and hence the decision to start with a chapter on anatomy and physiology. By understanding the usual structure and function of the body's organs, it will help gain an insight into the dysfunction of organs discussed later in the book.

Not only do nurses need to know the basics, they also need to have sufficient information to assist them as their roles develop within the speciality. As their roles expand with the erosion of medico/nursing boundaries, nurses need to understand the reasoning behind their individual actions and responsibilities. The nurse ordering investigations needs to have sufficient information to allow basic interpretation of results following the investigative request and, indeed, the need to refer onwards as appropriate.

It is for these reasons that a separate chapter has been allocated to urological investigations. This provides a quick reference section for nurses, allowing them to read about various tests and procedures, without wading through the main text. Also, some investigations are required in a number of conditions. Chapter 2 immediately cuts down the need for discussion in individual chapters, leaving more opportunity to discuss treatments and nursing procedures within the relevant text.

Chapters 4 to 8 are arranged in a systematic way, using the structures of the genitourinary tract as their guide. It is easiest to work with the 'top-down' approach, and therefore start with the kidney and ureters. This is then followed by chapters concerning the remaining structures, i.e. the bladder, prostate, penis and urethra, and the testicle. These chapters deal with dysfunction and treatment of conditions associated with each organ. All of them provide detail of nursing care and the psychological needs of the patient.

Some areas of urology are more specialized than others, needing extra care or a specialized approach. This is reflected in the decision to create specialist chapters concerning paediatric disorders (Chapter 3), gender reassignment (Chapter 9) and erectile dysfunction (Chapter 10). Each of these is a subspeciality within the speciality of urology, and thus their importance is not overlooked within the main text.

The newly qualified nurse and, indeed, the experienced nurse may well feel confused by some of the words or terms used in urology. For a point of easy reference, and to aid with speed of delivery of information there is a comprehensive glossary at the end of the book. This will allow nurses in the clinical setting to look up information quickly.

The book's main priority is to provide the latest information, in the right amount of detail, at the quickest reference rate possible. This book is designed in a systematic way to aid delivery of these needs.

Urinary catheters are used widely within the speciality, for a variety of reasons, and Chapter 12 discusses their design and selection in detail.

Patient empowerment and education are major issues for the new millennium – promoting partnerships in care delivery. Chapter 12 is dedicated to these issues, and also to the need for effective, efficient documentation of this collaborative care.

Chapter 1
Anatomy and physiology

Gaynor Bond

Urological nursing focuses on two systems. The first is the urinary system, which is one of the body's excretory systems. One of its main functions is to remove waste products from the blood and eliminate them from the body; its other functions include regulating the volume of body fluids and balancing the pH and electrolyte composition of these fluids.

Although the main focus of urological nursing is the urinary system, certain aspects of a second system – the male reproductive system – need to be explored as these systems work interdependently to maintain a balance, or homeostasis.

Structure of the urinary system

The urinary system is made up of the following components:

- two kidneys: these organs extract wastes from the blood and balance body fluids. They are also the organs of excretion that form urine
- two ureters: tubes which convey the urine from the kidneys to the urinary bladder
- one urinary bladder: a reservoir that collects and temporarily stores the urine
- one urethra: a tube that discharges urine from the bladder to the outside of the body for elimination.

Location of the kidneys

The kidneys are reddish coloured organs shaped like kidney beans. On average, each one measures about 10–12 cm in length, 0.5–1.5 cm in width and 2.5 cm in thickness. They are located against the muscles of the back in the upper abdomen, one on each side of the vertebral column, behind the peritoneum and below the diaphragm. They are protected by the lower ribs and the rib cartilages. They are embedded in, and held in position by, a mass of fat, and both the kidney and the renal fat are enclosed in a sheath of fibroelastic tissue (renal fascia). As they are positioned behind the peritoneal lining of the abdominal cavity they are said to be in the retroperitoneal space. Other retroperitoneal structures include the ureters and the adrenal (suprarenal) glands.

The blood supply to the kidney is brought by a short branch of the abdominal aorta called the renal artery. After entering the kidney, the renal artery subdivides into smaller and smaller branches, which eventually make contact with the functional units of the kidney, the nephrons. Blood leaves the kidney in vessels that finally merge to form the renal vein. The renal vein carries the blood into the inferior vena cava for return to the heart. The right kidney is slightly lower than the left because the liver occupies a large area on the right side.

Organs associated with the kidneys

As the kidneys lie on either side of the vertebral column, each is associated with a different group of structures.

Right kidney

- Superiorly – the right adrenal gland.
- Anteriorly – the right lobe of the liver, the duodenum and the right colic flexure.
- Posteriorly – the diaphragm and the muscles of the posterior abdominal wall.

Left kidney

- Superiorly – the left adrenal gland.
- Anteriorly – the spleen, stomach, pancreas, jejunum and left colic flexure.

- Posteriorly – the diaphragm and the muscles of the posterior abdominal wall.

Structure of the kidney

The kidney's concave medial border faces the vertebral column. Near the centre of the concave border is a notch called the hilus, through which the ureter leaves the kidney. Blood and lymphatic vessels and nerves also enter and exit the kidney through the hilus. The hilus is the entrance to a cavity in the kidney called the renal sinus.

There are three layers of tissue surrounding each kidney:

1. Renal capsule: the innermost layer, which is a smooth, transparent, fibrous membrane that is continuous with the outer coat of the ureter of the hilus. It serves as a barrier against trauma and the spread of infection to the kidney.
2. Adipose capsule: the middle layer, which is a mass of fatty tissue surrounding the renal capsule. This layer also protects the kidney from trauma and holds it firmly in place within the abdominal cavity.
3. Renal fascia: the outermost layer, which is a thin layer of dense, irregular connective tissue that anchors the kidney to its surrounding structures and to the abdominal wall.

The kidney is divided into three regions: the renal cortex, the renal medulla and the renal pelvis. The renal cortex is the reddish coloured outer portion of the kidney. The inner, reddish brown region is called the renal medulla, and it contains the tubes that collect urine. These tubes form between eight and 18 cone-shaped structures called renal pyramids. They appear striped, due to the presence of straight tubules and blood vessels. The face of each pyramid faces the cortex, and their apexes, called renal papillae, point towards the centre of the kidney. The cortex is a smooth textured area extending from the renal capsule to the bases of the pyramids and into the spaces between them. It is divided into an outer cortical zone and an inner juxtamedullary zone. Portions of the cortex extend between renal pyramids to form the renal columns.

Together, the cortex and the renal pyramids constitute the parenchyma (functional portion) of the kidney. Structurally, the parenchyma of each kidney consists of about 1 million microscopic structures called nephrons.

In the renal sinus of the kidney is a large cavity called the renal pelvis. The edge of the pelvis contains cup-like extensions called major and minor calyces. There are two or three major calyces and between eight and 18 minor calyces. Each minor calyx receives urine from collecting ducts of one pyramid and delivers urine to a major calyx. The urine then drains from the major calyces into the renal pelvis and out through the ureter to the urinary bladder.

The kidney is a glandular organ, that is, most of the tissue is epithelium with just enough connective tissue to serve as a framework. The basic unit of the kidney, where the work is actually done, is the nephron. The nephron is a tiny coiled tube with a bulb at one end. This bulb, called 'Bowman's capsule', surrounds a cluster of capillaries called the glomerulus. A small blood vessel, called the afferent arteriole, supplies the glomerulus with blood; another small vessel, called the efferent arteriole, carries blood from the glomerulus to the capillaries surrounding the coiled tube of the nephron. As these capillaries surround the tube, they are called the peritubular capillaries.

The tubular part of the nephron consists of several portions. The coiled portion leading from Bowman's capsule is called the proximal convoluted tubule and the coiled portion at the other end is called the distal convoluted tubule. Between these two coiled portions is the loop of Henle. The distal convoluted tubule curls back towards the glomerulus between the afferent and efferent arterioles. At the point at which the distal tubule contacts the arterioles, there are specialized glandular cells that form the juxtaglomerular apparatus.

The glomerulus, Bowman's capsule, and the proximal and distal convoluted tubules of most nephrons are within the renal cortex. The loops of Henle extend varying distances into the medulla. The distal end of each tubule empties into a collecting tubule, which then continues through the medulla towards the renal pelvis.

Nephrons have three basic functions – filtration, reabsorption and secretion.

Functions of the kidney

The kidneys are involved in the following processes:

- excretion of unwanted substances, such as waste products from cell metabolism, excess salts and toxins
- maintenance of water balance
- regulation of acid/base balance
- production of hormones, including renin, which is important in the regulation of blood pressure.

The kidneys form urine, which passes through the ureters to the bladder for excretion. The composition of urine reflects the activities of the nephrons in the maintenance of homeostatis. Waste products of protein metabolism are excreted, electrolyte balance is maintained and the acid/base balance is influenced by the excretion of hydrogen ions. There are three phases in the formation of urine:

- simple filtration
- selective reabsorption
- secretion.

The process of urine formation begins in the glomerulus and Bowman's capsule. Simple filtration takes place through the semipermeable walls of the glomerulus and glomerular capsule. Water and a large number of small molecules pass through, some of which are reabsorbed later. Blood cells, plasma proteins and other large molecules are unable to filter through and remain in the capillaries.

Because the diameter of the afferent arteriole is slightly larger than that of the efferent arteriole, blood can enter the glomerulus more rapidly than it can leave. Thus, the pressure of the blood in the glomerulus is about three or four times higher than it is in other body capillaries. As a result of this increased pressure, materials are constantly being 'squeezed' out of the blood into Bowman's capsule. This process is known as glomerular filtration. The fluid that enters Bowman's capsule, called glomerular filtrate, begins the journey along the tubular system of the nephron. In addition to water and the normal soluble substances in the blood, other substances, such as drugs, may also be filtered and become part of the glomerular filtrate (Figure 1.1).

About 180 litres of dilute filtrate are formed each day by the two kidneys. Of this, 1–1.5 litres are excreted as urine. The difference in volume and concentration is due to selective reabsorption of some constituents of the filtrate and secretion by tubular cells of others (Table 1.1).

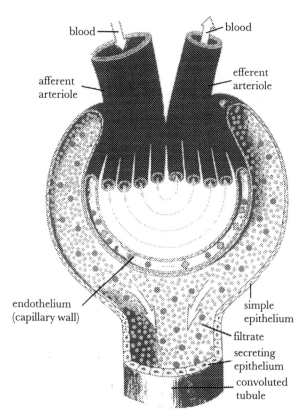

Diagram showing the process of filtration in the formation of urine. The high pressure inside the capillaries of the glomerulus forces the dissolved substances (but not plasma proteins) and water into the space inside the Bowman's capsule. The smaller calibre of the vessel as compared with that of the larger afferent vessel causes this pressure.

Figure 1.1 Urine formation.

Selective reabsorption is the process by which the composition and volume of glomerular filtrate are altered as it passes through the convoluted tubules, the loop of Henle and the collecting tubule. The purpose of this process is to reabsorb those filtrate constituents needed by the body, such as water, nutrients and ions, to maintain fluid and electrolyte balance and blood alkalinity.

Some constituents of glomerular filtrate do not normally appear in the urine because they are completely reabsorbed unless they are present in blood in excessive quantities. The kidney's maximum capacity for reabsorption of a substance is the transport maximum.

Table 1.1 Selective filtration

Blood constituents in glomerular filtrate	Blood constituents remaining in the glomerulus
Water	Leukocytes
Mineral salts	Erythrocytes
Amino acids	Platelets
Keto acids	Blood proteins
Glucose	
Hormones	
Urea	
Uric acid	
Toxins	
Drugs	

For example, normal blood glucose level is 2.5–5.3 mmol/l (45–95 mg/100 ml); if the level rises above the transport maximum of about 9 mmol/l (160 mg/100ml) glucose appears in the urine because the mechanism for active transfer out of the tubules is overloaded.

The transport maximum of some substances varies according to the body's need for them at the time, i.e. in order to maintain homeostasis. In some cases reabsorption is regulated by hormones:

- Parathryn from the parathyroid glands and calcitonin from the thyroid gland together regulate the reabsorption of calcium and phosphate.
- Antidiuretic hormone (ADH) from the posterior lobe of the pituitary gland affects the permeability of the distal convoluted tubules and collecting tubules, regulating water and reabsorption.
- Aldosterone secreted by the cortex of the adrenal gland influences the reabsorption of sodium and the excretion of potassium.

Waste products, such as urea and uric acid, are reabsorbed in very small amounts only. Substances that are not normal blood constituents are not reabsorbed. If the blood passes through the glomerulus too quickly for filtration to clear such substances from the blood, the tubules secrete them into the filtrate. Substances of no physiological significance are sometimes injected into the body to evaluate the kidney's excretory efficiency.

Secretion

Filtrate is produced as the blood flows through the glomerulus. Substances not required and foreign materials, e.g. drugs, may not be cleared from the blood by filtration because of the short time the blood remains in the glomerulus. Such substances are cleared by secretion into the convoluted tubules and passed from the body in the urine.

Urine is amber in colour due to the presence of urobilin, a bile pigment altered in the intestine, reabsorbed then excreted by the kidneys. The specific gravity of urine is between 1020 and 1030, and the reaction is acid. The amount of urine secreted and the specific gravity vary according to the fluid intake and the amount of solute excreted. During sleep and muscular exercise urine production is decreased.

Concentration of urine

Water is taken into the body through the alimentary tract and a small amount is formed by the metabolic processes. It is excreted in saturated expired air, as a constituent of the faeces, through the skin as sweat and as the main constituent of urine (Table 1.2). The amount lost in expired air and in the faeces is fairly constant and the amount of sweat produced is associated with the maintenance of normal body temperature.

Table 1.2 Composition of urine

Component	Amount
Water	96%
Urea	2%
Uric acid	
Creatinine	
Ammonia	
Sodium	
Potassium	2%
Chloride	
Phosphates	
Sulphates	
Oxalates	

The balance between fluid intake and output is controlled by the kidneys. The minimum urinary output, consistent with the essential removal of waste material is about 500 ml per day. The amount produced in excess of this is controlled mainly by antidiuretic hormone (ADH) released into the blood by the posterior lobe of the pituitary gland.

The concentrating mechanism is called the 'counter current mechanism', because it involves fluid travelling in opposite directions within the loop of Henle. As the filtrate passes through the loop of Henle, salts, especially sodium, are actively pumped out by the cells of the nephron, with the result that the interstitial fluid of the medulla becomes increasingly concentrated. Because the nephron is not very permeable to water at this point, the fluid within the nephron becomes increasingly dilute. As the fluid passes through the distal convoluted tubule and the collecting tubule, and then out of the kidney, water is drawn out by the concentrated fluids around the nephron and returned to the blood, thus reducing the volume of the urine. The role of ADH is to make the walls of the distal convoluted tubule and collecting tubule more permeable to water so that more water will be reabsorbed and less will be excreted in the urine. The release of ADH is regulated by a feedback system (Figure 1.2). As the blood becomes more concentrated, the hypothalamus causes more ADH to be released from the posterior pituitary; as the blood becomes more dilute, less ADH is released. In diabetes insipidus there is inadequate secretion of ADH from the hypothalamus, which results in the elimination of large amounts of very dilute urine, and excessive thirst.

Electrolyte balance

A change in the concentration of electrolytes in the body fluids may be due to a change in the amount of water or electrolytes. There are several methods of maintaining the balance between water and electrolyte concentration.

Sodium is the most common cation (positively charged ion) in extracellular fluid and potassium is the most common intracellular cation. Sodium is a constituent of almost all foods and is often added to food. This means that sodium intake is usually in excess of the body's needs. It is excreted mainly in urine and sweat.

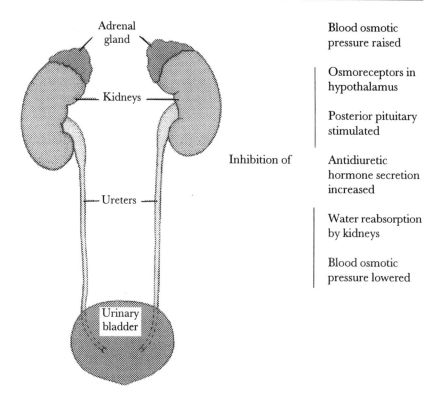

Adrenal
gland

Kidneys

Ureters

Urinary
bladder

Inhibition of

Blood osmotic
pressure raised

Osmoreceptors in
hypothalamus

Posterior pituitary
stimulated

Antidiuretic
hormone secretion
increased

Water reabsorption
by kidneys

Blood osmotic
pressure lowered

Figure 1.2 Feedback mechanism for the control of antidiuretic hormone (ADH) secretion.

Sodium is a normal constituent of urine and the amount excreted is regulated by the hormone aldosterone, secreted by the cortex of the adrenal gland (suprarenal gland). Cells in the afferent arteriole of the nephron are stimulated to produce the enzyme renin by sympathetic nerves or by low arteriole blood pressure. Renin converts angiotensinogen, produced by the liver, to angiotensin, which stimulates the adrenal gland to secrete aldosterone. Water is reabsorbed with sodium and together they increase the blood volume, leading to reduced renin secretion. When sodium reabsorption is increased, potassium excretion is increased, indirectly reducing intracellular potassium concentration (Figure 1.3). The amount of sodium excreted in sweat is insignificant, except when sweating is excessive. Normally the renal mechanism described maintains the cation concentration within physiological limits. When excessive sweating is sustained, acclimatization occurs in about 7 to 10 days and the amount of electrolyte lost in sweat is reduced.

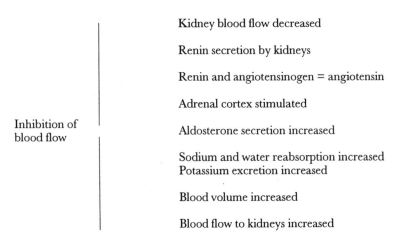

Kidney blood flow decreased

Renin secretion by kidneys

Renin and angiotensinogen = angiotensin

Adrenal cortex stimulated

Inhibition of blood flow

Aldosterone secretion increased

Sodium and water reabsorption increased
Potassium excretion increased

Blood volume increased

Blood flow to kidneys increased

Figure 1.3 Relationship between renal blood flow and selective reabsorption by the nephron.

Sodium and potassium occur in high concentrations in digestive juices – sodium in gastric juice and potassium in pancreatic and intestinal juice. Normally these ions are reabsorbed by the colon, but following acute or prolonged diarrhoea they may be excreted in large quantities, with resultant electrolyte imbalance.

To maintain the normal blood pH, hydrogen ions are secreted by the cells of the convoluted tubules and are excreted in the urine. They are secreted in combination with bicarbonate as carbonic acid, with ammonia as ammonium chloride and with hydrogen phosphate as dihydrogen phosphate. The normal pH of urine varies from 4.5 to 7.8 depending on diet, time of day and a number of other factors.

The adrenal glands

The adrenals, or suprarenals, are two small glands located above the kidneys. Each adrenal gland has two parts, which act as separate glands. The inner area is called the medulla and the outer portion is called the cortex. Both produce hormones (Table 1.3).

Hormones from the adrenal medulla

The hormones produced by the adrenal medulla are released in response to stimulation by the sympathetic nervous system. The principal hormone is epinephrine, also called adrenaline. Another hormone, called norepinephrine, is also produced. It is closely related chemically to epinephrine and is similar but not identical in

Table 1.3 The function of the adrenal glands

Gland	Hormone	Principal function
Adrenal medulla	Epinephrine and norepinephrine	Increases blood pressure and heart rate; activates cells influenced by sympathetic nervous system plus many not affected by sympathetic nerves
Adrenal cortex	Cortisol (95% of glucocorticoids)	Aids in metabolism of carbohydrates, proteins and fats; active during stress
	Aldosterone (95% of mineralocorticoids)	Aids in the regulation of electrolytes and water balance
	Sex hormones	May influence secondary sexual characteristics in males

its actions. These are referred to as the 'fight or flight' hormones because of their effects during emergency situations. Some of these effects are as follows:

- Stimulation of the involuntary muscle in the walls of the arterioles, causing these muscles to contract and blood pressure to rise.
- Conversion of the glycogen stored in the liver into glucose. The glucose enters the blood and is delivered to the voluntary muscles, permitting them to do an extraordinary amount of work.
- Increase in heart rate.
- Increase in the metabolic rate of body cells.
- Dilation of the bronchioles, through relaxation of the smooth muscle of their walls.

Hormones from the adrenal cortex

There are three main groups of hormones secreted by the adrenal cortex.

1. Glucocorticoids maintain the carbohydrate reserve of the body by controlling the conversion of amino acids into sugar instead of

protein. These hormones are produced in larger than normal amounts in times of stress and so aid the body in responding to unfavourable conditions. They have the ability to suppress the inflammatory response and are often administered as medication for this purpose. A major hormone of this group is cortisol, which is also called hydrocortisone.

2. Mineralocorticoids are important in the regulation of electrolyte balance. They control the reabsorption of sodium and the secretion of potassium by the kidney tubules. The major hormone of this group is aldosterone.

3. Sex hormones are normally secreted, but in small amounts. Their effects on the body are slight.

Location of the ureters

There are two ureters – one for each kidney – which carry urine from the kidneys to the urinary bladder. Each ureter is 25–30 cm in length, with a diameter of about 3 mm, and is an extension of the pelvis of the kidney. Like the kidneys the ureters are retroperitoneal in placement. The ureters enter the urinary bladder obliquely (at an angle) from the posterior aspect (Figure 1.4).

The ureters enter the bladder through an oblique tunnel that functions as a valve, preventing backflow of urine into the ureters during bladder contraction. As the urinary bladder fills with urine, pressure inside compresses the ureteral openings and prevents back up of urine into the ureters.

Structure of the ureters

The wall of the ureters comprises three layers of tissue:

1. An outer covering of fibrous tissue, continuous with the fibrous capsule of the kidney.
2. A middle, muscular layer consisting of interlacing muscle fibres that form a syncytium spiralling around the ureter, some in clockwise and some in anticlockwise directions, and an additional outer longitudinal layer in the lower third.
3. An inner layer of transitional epithelium.

Function of the ureters

The principal function of the ureters is to transport urine from the

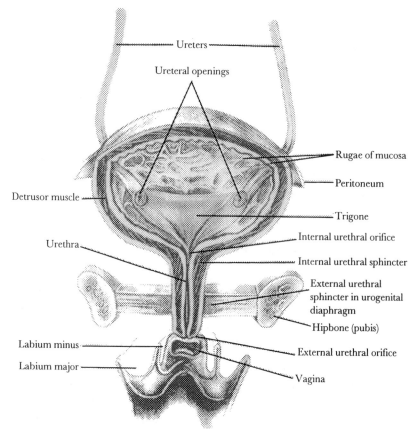

Figure 1.4 Coronal section, viewed from anterior.

renal pelvis into the urinary bladder. Peristaltic contraction of the muscular walls pushes urine towards the bladder, but hydrostatic pressure and gravity also contribute. The waves of contraction originate in a pacemaker in the minor calyces. Peristaltic waves occur at about 10 second intervals, sending little spurts of urine into the bladder.

The urinary bladder

Location of the urinary bladder

The urinary bladder is a reservoir for urine. When it is empty, it is situated below the parietal peritoneum and behind the pubic joint. In the male, it is directly anterior to the rectum. In the female, it is anterior to the vagina and inferior to the uterus. When the urinary bladder is filled, it pushes the peritoneum upwards and may extend well into the abdominal cavity. It is a freely movable organ held in position by folds of the peritoneum. In general, bladder capacity is smaller in females because the uterus occupies space just above the bladder.

Organs associated with the bladder

In the female

- Anteriorly – the symphysis pubis.
- Posteriorly – the uterus and upper part of the vagina.
- Superiorly – the small intestine.
- Inferiorly – the urethra and the muscles forming the pelvic floor.

In the male

- Anteriorly – the symphysis pubis.
- Posteriorly – the rectum and seminal vesicles.
- Superiorly – the small intestine.
- Inferiorly – the urethra and prostate gland.

Structure of the urinary bladder

The empty bladder is roughly pear-shaped, but it becomes more oval as it fills with urine. In the floor of the urinary bladder is a small triangular area, the trigone. The two posterior corners of the trigone contain the two ureteral openings and the opening into the urethra (internal urethral orifice) lies in the anterior corner. Because its mucosa is firmly bound to the muscularis, the trigone has a smooth appearance.

The bladder wall has three layers:

1. The outer layer of loose connective tissue, containing blood and lymphatic vessels and nerves.
2. The middle layer, consisting of a mass of interlacing smooth muscle fibres and elastic tissue loosely arranged in three layers.
3. The lining of transitional epithelium.

When the bladder is empty or contracted the inner lining is arranged in folds, which gradually disappear as the bladder fills.

Functions of the bladder

Urine is expelled from the bladder in an act called micturition, commonly known as urination or voiding. Near the outlet of the bladder, a circle of smooth muscle forms the internal sphincter, which contracts to prevent emptying. The average capacity of the urinary bladder is 700–800 ml. When the amount of urine present exceeds 200–400 ml, stretch receptors in the wall transmit nerve impulses to the lower part of the spinal chord. From there, motor impulses are sent out to the bladder musculature and the organ is emptied. In the infant this emptying is automatic (a reflex action). As a child matures, higher brain centres gain control over the reflex action and over a voluntary external sphincter that is located below the internal sphincter and certain muscles of the urogenital (pelvic) diaphragm. The time of urination can be voluntarily controlled unless the bladder becomes too full.

The urethra

Location of the urethra

The urethra is a tube leading from the floor of the urinary bladder to the exterior of the body. In females it lies directly posterior to the pubic symphysis and is in front of the anterior wall of the vagina. Its undilated diameter is about 6 mm, and it is approximately 3.8 cm in length. The female urethra is directed obiquely, inferiorly and anteriorly. The opening of the urethra to the exterior, the external urethral orifice, is located between the clitoris and vaginal opening.

In males, the urethra is about 20 cm long. Immediately below the urinary bladder it passes vertically through the prostate gland (prostatic urethra), then pierces the urogenital diaphragm (membranous urethra), and finally pierces the penis (spongy urethra) and takes a curved course through the body.

Structure of the urethra

The wall of the urethra comprises three layers of tissue:

1. A muscular layer which is continuous with that of the bladder. At its origin is an internal sphincter, composed mainly of elastic tissue and smooth muscle fibres, under autonomic control. Near the external urethral orifice the smooth muscle is replaced by striated muscle which forms the external sphincter, under voluntary control.
2. A thin, spongy coat containing large numbers of blood vessels.

3. A lining of mucous membrane continuous with that of the bladder in the upper part of the urethra. The lower part consists of stratified squamous epithelium, continuous externally with the skin of the vulva.

Function of the urethra

The urethra is the terminal portion of the urinary system. It serves as the passageway for discharging urine from the body. The male urethra also serves as the duct through which reproductive fluid (semen) is discharged from the body.

The male reproductive system

The prostate gland

The prostate gland is a single, doughnut-shaped gland about the size of a chestnut. It lies immediately below the urinary bladder, where it surrounds the superior portion of the urethra. Ducts from the prostate secrete a milky, slightly acidic fluid that contains citric acid and several enzymes, including fibrinolysin. Clotting enzymes cause the fibrinogen contributed by the seminal vesicles to coagulate the semen shortly after ejaculation. Fibrinolysin subsequently breaks down the clot. These secretions enter the prostatic urethra through many prostatic ducts. They make up about 25% of the volume of semen and contribute to sperm motility and viability. The prostate gland is also supplied with muscular tissue, which upon signal from the nervous system contracts to aid in the expulsion of the semen from the body. The prostate gland slowly increases in size from birth to puberty, and then a rapid growth spurt occurs. The size attained by the third decade remains stable until about age 45, when further enlargement may occur and lead to a number of disorders, such as benign enlargement, prostatic cancer and retention of urine due to outflow obstruction.

The testicles

The testes or testicles are the male reproductive glands and are the equivalent of the ovaries in the female. The testicles are paired, oval glands measuring about 5 cm in length and 2.5 cm in diameter (Figure 1.5). Each weighs between 10 and 15 g. They are normally located

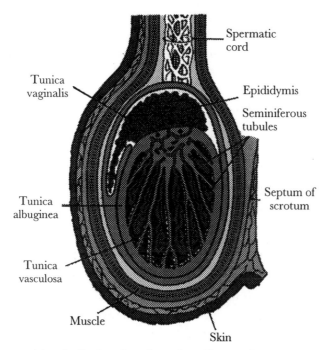

Spermatic cord

Tunica vaginalis

Epididymis

Seminiferous tubules

Tunica albuginea

Septum of scrotum

Tunica vasculosa

Muscle

Skin

A longitudinal section of a testis and its coverings

Figure 1.5 The testicle.

outside the body proper, suspended between the thighs in a sac called the scrotum. During embryonic life the testes develop from the tissue near the kidney. A month or two before birth, the testes normally descend through the inguinal canal in the abdominal wall into the scrotum. Each testicle must descend completely if it is to function normally. In order to produce spermatozoa, the testicles must be kept at the temperature of the scrotum, which is lower than that of the abdominal cavity.

In each testis there are between 200 and 300 lobules and within each lobule there are one to four convoluted loops composed of germinal epithelial cells, called seminiferous tubules. Between the tubules there are groups of interstitial Leydig cells, which secrete the hormone testosterone. At the upper pole of the testis the tubules combine to form a tortuous tubule, the epididymis, which leaves the scrotum as the deferent duct in the spermatic cord. Blood and lymph vessels pass to the testes in the spermatic cords.

After being secreted by the testicles, testosterone is absorbed directly into the blood stream. This hormone has two functions. The first is maintenance of the reproductive structures, including the development of spermatozoa. The second involves the development of secondary sex characteristic traits that characterize males and females but are not directly concerned with reproduction. In males they include a deeper voice, broader shoulders, narrow hips, a greater percentage of muscle tissue and more body hair than is found in females.

Penis

The penis is used to introduce spermatozoa into the vagina and for expelling urine from the body. It is cylindrical in shape and consists of a body, root and glans penis (Figure 1.6).

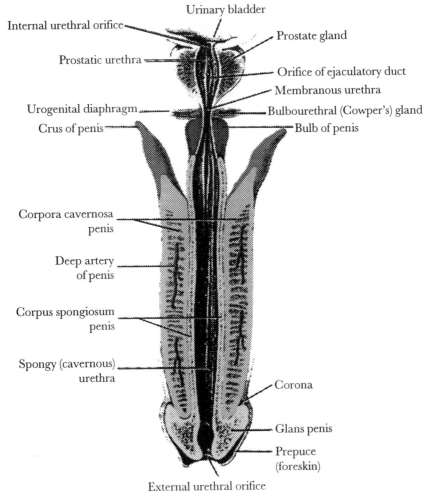

Urinary bladder

Internal urethral orifice

Prostate gland

Prostatic urethra

Orifice of ejaculatory duct

Membranous urethra

Urogenital diaphragm

Bulbourethral (Cowper's) gland

Crus of penis

Bulb of penis

Corpora cavernosa penis

Deep artery of penis

Corpus spongiosum penis

Spongy (cavernous) urethra

Corona

Glans penis

Prepuce (foreskin)

External urethral orifice

Figure 1.6 The penis.

The root lies in the perineum and the body surrounds the urethra. It is formed from three elongated masses of erectile tissue and involuntary muscle. The erectile tissue is supported by fibrous tissue and is covered with skin. It also has a rich blood supply.

The two lateral columns are called the corpora cavernosa and the column between them, containing the urethra, is the corpus spongiosum. At its tip it is expanded into a triangular structure known as the glans penis. Just above the glans the skin is folded upon itself and forms a movable double layer – the foreskin or prepuce. The distal urethra enlarges within the glans penis and forms a terminal slit-like opening, the external urethral orifice.

With sexual stimulation, which may be visual, tactile, auditory, olfactory or imaginative, the arteries supplying the penis dilate and large quantities of blood enter the blood sinuses. Expansion of these spaces compresses the veins draining the penis, so most entering blood is trapped. These vascular changes result in an erection, a parasympathetic reflex. The penis returns to its flaccid state when the arteries constrict and pressure on the veins is relieved. Ejaculation, the propulsion from the urethra to the exterior, is a sympathetic reflex. As part of the reflex, the smooth muscle sphincter at the base of the urinary bladder closes. Thus urine is not expelled during ejaculation and semen does not enter the urinary bladder.

Chapter 2
Urological investigations

LISA GRANT

This chapter provides a quick reference guide for some of the common investigations undertaken in urology. It is important that confidentiality, patient dignity and privacy are recognized and upheld in all of the procedures described below.

Biopsies

A biopsy is a sample of tissue taken from the patient, under either general or local anaesthetic. The tissue is then sent for diagnostic study. Reporting of results from biopsies can take some time and this can be a worrying period for the patient and his or her partner. Nurses need to be aware of this potential anxiety and possible mood changes of the patient.

The various biopsies taken in urology may include:

- *Bladder biopsy*: this is usually performed during a cystoscopy. The tissue sample is obtained by using either forceps or a resectoscope.
- *Testicular biopsy*: this is usually performed when investigating infertility. The tissue is obtained when making an incision into the tunica albuginea. When a tumour is suspected, a biopsy of the affected testicle is not normally taken. In this instance an orchidectomy is usually performed – thus excising the tumour. However, biopsy of the unaffected testicle is often performed at the time of the orchidectomy to verify that there has been no spread of the disease.

- *Prostate biopsy:* these are often taken with the purpose of confirming the diagnosis of malignant disease of the prostate, when other investigations have not been able to confirm the diagnosis. The biopsy can be taken either by open operation through the perineum or retropubic space, or through the anterior wall of the rectum. Antibiotic cover is often provided to prevent subsequent bacteraemia.

Endoscopic procedures

Cystoscopy and flexiscope procedure

This procedure can be carried out under general or local anaesthetic, depending on the physical condition of the patient. It allows an interior view of the bladder using either a rigid cystoscope when under general anaesthetic or a flexible cystoscope when under local.

The procedure allows the surgeon to take biopsies where suspicious lesions are present. The common indicators for this procedure include presentation with haematuria or recurrent urinary tract infections.

General anaesthetic

The patient will be kept free from fluids and diet for approximately seven hours preoperatively. Postoperatively, the patient should be encouraged to drink so that he or she is able to pass urine. This needs to be measured each time the patient voids, and documented so that any abnormalities can be detected.

The patient should be advised that their urine may contain some blood. This can be due to trauma experienced when the scope is inserted, and may come from the bladder or urethra. Following discharge, they should be advised to inform their GP if this continues.

Local anaesthetic

There is no restriction on fluid or dietary intake prior to this procedure. A light diet is advised to keep the bowel free from faeces to prevent any obstruction when the cystoscope is inserted.

Post-procedure, the patient should be encouraged to void as soon as possible. He or she should be encouraged to drink plenty of fluids, and on discharge home should be given the same advice as patients who have had a general anaesthetic. It may be preferable for the information on discharge to be in written format.

Check cystoscopies

These are initially carried out every three months, to look for regrowth following treatment of a bladder tumour. They are eventually spread over a longer period, i.e. six-monthly to 12-monthly depending on the results of the cystoscopy. The patient will have these checkups for at least a 10-year period following initial diagnosis.

Digital rectal examination

A digital rectal examination can often detect an enlarged prostate. The practitioner feels its size shape and texture. An enlarged smooth prostate tends to indicate benign growth, whereas a lumpy, nodular texture tends to indicate malignant growth.

If the prostate is enlarged, it may cause outflow obstruction. However, size is not specifically related to outflow obstruction, and this may be misleading. Other procedures including urinary flow rate test and residual volume may also be required.

Prior to the examination, the patient should be advised to have a light diet and he should be encouraged to open his bowels prior to the procedure. The patient is asked to lie on his left lateral side with his knees drawn to his chest.

After the examination, he may eat and drink as normal.

Urethroscopy

The principles of urethroscopy are the same as those of cystoscopy. However, the focus of the examination is the urethra.

A urethroscope is inserted (usually under general anaesthetic) for the visual examination of any suspicious lesions. Pre- and postoperative care are the same as for cystoscopy.

Flow rate test

The urinary flow rate test measures the rate at which urine is emptied from the urinary bladder, including time taken, volume voided and the speed in millimetres per second. This procedure can establish if there is any outflow obstruction, which may indicate an enlarged prostate, tight bladder neck or urethral stricture.

Prior to the procedure, the patient is required to fill his or her bladder, drinking between one and one and a half litres of water or other liquid. When the patient feels the need to void, he or she is asked to do so into a funnel connected to a flow rate machine.

There are two types of flow rate machine: digital and graph readings. The digital machine has four main readings: volume, peak flow, mean flow, and voiding time. The graph machine, however draws out a graph of the voiding pattern with squares on the graph representing amount voided on the vertical scale and time taken on the horizontal scale.

Discussion surrounds the number of times a flow rate should be performed for accuracy. Current thought is that three should be the optimum frequency, in order to ensure an accurate diagnosis.

Intravenous urogram (IVU, formerly IVP)

An IVU study involves an intravenous injection of an iodine contrast medium, which will subsequently allow X-rays of the bladder, kidneys and ureters to be taken. This investigation will detect the absence of a kidney, irregularities of the bladder, and any possible obstruction in either the kidney or the ureter.

Prior to the procedure, the patient should be prescribed a laxative so that the bowel is emptied and clear, accurate pictures can be obtained.

Fluids should be restricted prior to the examination – up to 500 ml of fluid may be taken up to two hours prior to the procedure. A light meal can be taken during this time also. Ideally, a diabetic patient should have the procedure performed as early in the morning as possible so that restrictions on dietary intake are kept to a minimum.

Patients allergic to iodine should not undergo IVU. Asthmatic patients require steroid cover pre- and post-procedure because of the contrast medium used.

Kidney, ureter and bladder X-ray (KUB)

This imaging process is a plain film which visualizes the abdomen and surveys the urinary tract. It also determines the size, shape and placement of the urological structures, therefore detecting any abnormalities.

The procedure can be used in the initial investigation of a patient's complaint or symptom, or it may be used in conjunction with other tests.

A mild laxative may be prescribed prior to the procedure to clear out the bowel in order to give a clearer picture. Usually no preparation is needed.

The patient should be informed about the procedure, as with any other X-ray. This should include information about the exposure to some radiation and the effects of this, making sure that anyone who is or suspects that she may be pregnant does not undergo the procedure.

Nuclear imaging

Bone scan

A bone scan is conducted when either a lesion or tumour has been found. Patients with prostate cancer are scanned due to the high probability of widespread metastases. This scan is used in the assessment of patients with suspected bony metastases and the detection of functional change due to metabolic bone disease.

The scan is a simple imaging process, enabling pictures of the skeletal system to be obtained. A radioactive medium is injected into a vein following cannulation, and this then passes via the blood to the bones. After injection of the medium there is a waiting period of approximately three hours, during which time the patient is advised to drink plenty of fluids. This will help to obtain clear images with the scan.

No preparation is required prior to this procedure. The patient may also eat and drink normally after the scan.

Mag III renograms

This is a dynamic/static imaging process in the assessment of kidney function. An intravenous injection of TMAG3 is given, and then by use of a gamma camera, a quantitative estimation of function in each kidney is given. Patients are kept well hydrated during the process.

The images generated during this process are then constructed into a graph of function, i.e. the renogram is constructed. The normal renogram is in three parts: the vascular phase; a rise caused by the secretory action of the kidney; and a decrease as the urine, which is radioactive, drains from the kidney.

There is no preparation prior to this procedure, and the patient may eat and drink normally.

Renal arteriogram

Arteriograms show the interior of arteries – in this case, the arteries of the kidney. This procedure is usually carried out after an IVU, where renal swelling has been shown. The arteriogram allows a more accurate diagnosis due to the fact that the arteries show a distinctive appearance if they are near to a cyst or tumour.

Prior to the procedure, the patient is kept nil by mouth and a written consent form is needed. The patient is gowned as for theatre, and the groin area needs to be shaved (as per local protocol). The radiologist introduces a large needle into the femoral artery, and a catheter is threaded along this needle into the renal artery. Injecting a contrast medium into the catheter outlines the arterial tree and X-ray pictures can be taken.

Post-procedure, pressure is maintained over the puncture site of the femoral artery, and the patient should be advised to lie flat for four to six hours. Vital signs should be recorded every 15 minutes for half an hour, then hourly until a satisfactory medium is given.

Routine testing of urine

On admission to hospital, the patient's urine should be tested at ward level. The routine testing of urine can rule out primary infection, which could indicate possible obstruction or tumour necrosis. It allows staff to detect if the patient has any blood in his or her urine, which may indicate tumour growth.

Catheter specimens

Catheter specimens are taken primarily to rule out infection. The catheter sample should be taken using a sterile needle and syringe, using aseptic technique, to minimize the risk of infection.

Most catheter bags have a sample port (normally consisting of a self-sealing rubber band around the tubing) to allow for aspiration of the urine sample.

Cytology specimens

The patient is asked to void the whole volume of his or her bladder into a bedpan or urinal. This whole sample is then sent to the laboratory for analysis, with the aim of identifying tumour cells.

A cytology specimen should be collected from any patient presenting with haematuria because of the risk of tumour cells being present.

Mid-stream specimens

This procedure involves taking a sample of urine mid-stream when voiding. Three specimens may be taken: first, when a patient initially starts to void; mid-stream; and at the end. The rationale behind this is the location of the source of infection or the source of haematuria being voided. These specimens are sent for laboratory investigation.

Red blood cells found in the initial specimen of urine suggest bleeding from the anterior urethra; in mid-stream they suggest bleeding from the posterior urethra or bladder neck. Blood cells in all specimens will imply bleeding originates from any of these sites.

Residual volume ultrasound scan

This scan can be carried out at ward level, usually after the patient has undergone a flow rate test. It involves the use of a portable scanner to measure the amount of urine in the bladder using ultrasound waves. It allows staff to recognize if the patient is in retention, thus allowing appropriate medical intervention.

No preparation is needed prior to the procedure apart from asking the patient to void before the scan is performed.

The head of the scanner is placed on the patient's lower abdomen in the area of the bladder, using scanning gel to allow conduction of the ultrasound waves. The scanner head is then tilted in various directions until the residual volume is ascertained. A printout is then produced, showing the residual volume. This can be fixed into the casenotes. It is a quick procedure to undertake and gives relatively accurate results.

Residual volume catheterization

The indicators for this are as for residual volume ultrasound scanning. Some wards will not have access to a scanner, and therefore the patient needs to be catheterized to obtain the same results.

The patient is asked to void. Following this, a non-balloon catheter, such as a Nelaton catheter, is passed using aseptic technique. As the drainage starts to tail off, the catheter is slowly removed to allow maximum drainage. The volume drained is then measured and documented.

Ultrasound studies

An ultrasound is one of the first studies to be carried out when identifying any abnormalities in the ureters, kidneys or bladder. It involves light-frequency sound waves being transmitted through the skin and reflected by the internal organs and structures. These echoes then form a picture on screen, which can be examined for any abnormalities. An ultrasound can show cysts, tumours and infections, and is a safe technique to use.

For most ultrasound examinations no specific care is needed before the test. However, when scanning the kidneys patients should be advised to avoid fizzy drinks, which may cause wind. When scanning the bladder, patients are often required to drink until their bladder is full. This enables clearer pictures to be obtained.

Urodynamic studies

This is a broad term that refers to a series of diagnostic techniques with the aim of evaluating the process of micturition, when an individual presents with a voiding dysfunction. The most common technique in urology is that of cystometry.

The cystometrogram is a measure of bladder capacity and the recording of pressure during fluid intake and storage stages of micturition.

The bladder can be stretched by introducing varying volumes of fluid into it, and recording the pressure produced. A two-way catheter is inserted into the bladder, the bladder is emptied and the residual volume is measured. One limb of the catheter is connected to a reservoir of sterile fluid, and the other to a recording manometer.

Cystometry is a useful investigation but in some cases as much can be ascertained about an individual's bladder function by taking a careful history and examination.

Assessment of patients

Holism and nursing care

The need for holistic nursing care has been well established over the past 10–15 years. This is best represented by the fact that in the majority of settings, in both acute and continuing care, each team of nurses has adopted a model of nursing. This creates a corporate sense of caring with the same values and emphasis.

The models of nursing take account of the individual as a whole entity – not just a set of clinical conditions. An assessment should be made of the person, taking into consideration not just their physical problems but also any psychological issues or anxieties. Some cases within the urological setting may well be 'curable' by examining the psychological issues. The patient with stress-induced impotence is a prime example.

Nursing interventions are numerous and variable. Each individual has their own needs. These can only be met once an assessment has been made. Assessment is an ongoing process, and it is not a restricted, single moment.

Assessment in urology

To make an assessment of value, there needs to be an agreed criterion within an assessment tool. All patients should be measured against this tool, where appropriate, using standardized questions.

In some cases, a nationally agreed model may be used, such as the Colley Model for measuring continence, the International Prostate Symptom Score for prostatic symptoms or the Waterflow score for measuring pressure area risk. Each of these models will provide an indicator for the treatment plan to be offered to the patient.

Other cases will be measured using locally devised assessment models, such as in an impotence clinic where there may be no nationally agreed assessment method.

In all cases, the approach to assessment should be uniform in that particular setting, so that locally agreed protocols for treatment can be actioned. It is important to remember, though, that while the method of assessment is standardized and even compartmentalized, the patient is an individual and should be treated as such.

Routine preoperative care

Preparation for theatre will vary between different trusts. However, in most cases, there is a standard method of theatre preparation.

Usually, the patient is kept nil by mouth for a period of 6 hours preoperatively if a general anaesthetic is to be administered. Very often, this is interpreted as being from midnight the night before theatre if they are on a morning list and from 7 am if on an afternoon list. These parameters will vary according to the specific operation and the wishes of individual anaesthetists.

Prior to theatre the patient should shower or bathe in an antiseptic solution, and wear a theatre gown without any underwear. Hair grips and jewellery should be removed, and ideally this includes removal of rings. However, rings may be taped if the patient wishes. These items are removed in order to prevent burns from the theatre diathermy machines.

To give the patient a psychological boost, prostheses such as eyes, wigs and false teeth can frequently be left in situ until entering the anaesthetic room if the patient wishes. These items can be removed in theatre and replaced prior to the patient returning to the ward.

The patient should have signed a consent form preoperatively, and relevant blood samples, electrocardiograms (ECGs) and X-rays should all be present prior to the patient leaving the ward. The nurse should check that all of these are in order prior to transportation to theatre.

The patient should also be wearing a legible and correctly detailed name band. This should be checked against the casenotes immediately prior to the patient leaving the ward. The nurse should check that the patient knows about the operation he or she is going for (describing it as best as he or she can) before allowing him or her to leave the ward.

Chapter 3
Paediatric urology

CAROLINE BARROW

Congenital paediatric abnormalities of the urinary tract

First, a clear distinction needs to be made regarding organic and functional urological problems children may experience with continence. Congenital abnormalities of the urological system do exist for both boys and girls, and may lead to varying degrees of difficulties in attaining continence. However, many of the children who present to the urologist, GP or nephrologist with a history of day/night-time wetting will not have an underlying organic pathophysiology. Functional problems do exist and treatment regimes, including medication and biofeedback, exist to support these children and their families.

Common non-obstructed urological problems

Hypospadias

Hypospadias is a common anomaly in boys, with an incidence in the general population estimated at 3–4 per 1000 live births (Thomas and Barker 1997). Hypospadias is the result of a malformation, a failure of the urethral folds to fuse on the ventral aspect of the penis. The urethra opens ventrally anywhere from a few millimetres from the glans to as far back as the perineum. Furthermore, the penis may be deviated by chordee, which is fibrous tissue found anteriorly to the urethral orifice, causing ventral curvature of the penis (Dawson and

Whitfield 1996). The condition is non-obstructive and treatment should begin with referral to a urologist for assessment.

Treatment options are surgical, the rationale for surgery being indicated by the following:

- The abnormality is visible and is unacceptable to the family or child.
- The urinary stream is altered.
- Associated chordee and altered stream could lead to difficulties with later sexual function and ejaculation.

Surgical repair for hypospadias is commonly seen on paediatric urology wards and, following initial assessment in the outpatient setting, routine admission is arranged for when the child is approximately 18 months of age. The surgical approach is determined by the consultant urologist, but can be influenced by the position of the meatus, the position of the distal urethra, presence or absence of associated chordee, and the quality and size of the foreskin.

The literature suggests many operations for hypospadias repair, however, Magpi, Mathieu, Duckett and Onlay Island Flap repair are the most common one-stage repairs (Bullock et al. 1994). If a staged repair of hypospadias is needed, this may heighten family anxiety and the paediatric urological nurse needs to be mindful that additional support may be needed. A successful primary operation is always the aim of the diligent urologist. However, there is a small chance of a need for a further surgery due to complications such as stricture, fistula and breakdown of the distal urethra. These may be due to infection, tension, overlapping suture lines and skin flap ischaemia (Bullock et al. 1994).

Nursing issues

Preoperative information needs to be shared with the family, as aftercare following surgery may require the use of a catheter as a urethral stent to aid repair. Admission is usually on the day of surgery. The child often returns to the ward with an indwelling catheter and a dressing; silastic foam dressings are common in practice but not used universally. The catheter acts as a stent to aid urethra repair and stays in place for several days depending on the surgical approach undertaken. Antibiotic and anticholinergic medications are frequently administered while the catheter remains in place to minimize the risk of infection and bladder spasms.

Removal of the dressing is undertaken by a competent practitioner in the ward environment. The child will require analgesia, and diversional play therapy can be a significant factor in the easy removal of the dressing. It has been suggested that removal of the dressing for hypospadias repair is traumatic for the child and family (Rose 1992). The nurse needs to be diligent to promote effective communication with the child and family, offering explanation of actions, and to liaise with the medical team if strong analgesia is needed to calm the child before removing the dressing. Once the child is passing urine well he can go home with discharge instructions/information and a follow-up outpatient appointment with the consultant urologist.

Circumcision

The rationale for circumcision falls into one of three categories: religious, tradition and when medically indicated. The debate regarding the number of boys who actually need circumcision continues, with figures in some regions declining steadily (Rickwood 1989). Traditionally circumcision was suggested to minimize urinary infections and to prevent common foreskin problems in childhood and adulthood; however in the age of evidence-based medicine, traditional approaches to management need to be validated in practice (Rickwood 1992). During embryological development the foreskin grows forward over the glans, with no definitive separation. Therefore preputial 'adhesions' are normal, with spontaneous separation commencing distally around the time of birth and continuing during childhood (Rickwood 1992; Dawson and Whitfield 1996). Natural development suggests that ballooning of the foreskin is not uncommon and does not automatically necessitate surgical intervention. There are a small number of boys who develop a true phimosis and these will certainly need medical intervention. Balanitis xerotics obliterans is a non-infective aggressive fibrosis of the foreskin. The cause is unknown and the treatment is unquestionably circumcision.

Nursing issues

Although circumcision can be viewed as routine day-care surgery, it can carry a risk of complication. Serious bleeding is the most common complication; others include stenosis and partial amputation (Ozdemir 1997). Although none of these is common, nor is it an exhaustive list of complications, the nurse needs to be mindful that complications can arise and medical intervention should be sought if necessary.

Often, the most difficult task for the nurse is the removal of the dressing applied to the circumcised penis. Due to the flow of urine, dressings can frequently become dislodged and result in the penis becoming stuck to the nappy or underclothes. Promoting good hygiene and showers rather than baths may alleviate some discomfort and ease removal of dressings until such time as the penis is healed.

Undescended testis (cryptorchidism)

The incidence of undescended testis after the first year of life is somewhere between 1 and 2% of full-term male births. The incidence of undescended testis for the pre-term infant increases with early gestational age. Therefore birth weight and gestational maturity have a significant impact on the degree of incidence (Fonkalsrud 1996).

The testis develops on the posterior abdominal wall close to the mesonephric ridge and enters a dormant phase from the end of the first trimester. Around the seventh month of gestation, descent will begin down to the scrotal swellings, through an opening in the anterior abdominal wall. Failure of the processus vaginalis to close following transition of the testis may result in a hernia needing surgical intervention. If undescended testes are not treated, higher surrounding temperature leads to altered spermatogenesis in later life. Undescended testes are also at risk of malignant degeneration in later life and therefore even if they cannot be placed into the scrotum, orchidectomy should be considered after puberty (Dawson and Whitfield 1996). Psychological problems may be experienced in the adolescent or adult and prostheses are available to enhance physical appearance. Treatment is surgical and many centres offer day-case or overnight surgery.

Nursing issues

Parents may be anxious about future fertility and the nurse needs to have a basic understanding of the outcome from surgery being positive. While previously, bed rest was indicated for several days following surgery, this is no longer seen as necessary. Good hygiene should be promoted once the wound has healed, with the majority of centres using dissolvable sutures, thus negating the need for stitch removal.

Duplication of the upper urinary tract/ectopic ureter

Complete ureteral duplication occurs when two ureteral buds originate close together at the normal position on the mesonephric duct. The varying growth rates of the buds leads to varying degrees of duplication, such that only the pelvis and upper ureter may be involved; or a complete duplication may exist, with both ureters opening into the bladder; or with a duplication anywhere along the system.

Incidence of this type of abnormality is difficult to assess, as only those children or adults who present with symptoms are likely to need intervention, therefore potentially leaving a significant healthy number in the population. However, duplication can be familial and is more common in girls. Where both ureters enter the bladder then the duplication is complete with the ureter draining the upper pole inserted ectopically into the bladder or occasionally into the vagina or urethra in females, prostatic urethra or ejaculatory ducts in males (Cudow and Thomas 1997).

Girls with an ectopic ureter will complain of being permanently wet between otherwise normal voids. Dryness at night may be possible due to the pooling of urine in the abnormal system. Clinical detection of this anomaly can be difficult. Cystoscopy and a methylene blue test can be helpful. The aim of the methylene blue test is to fill the bladder with dye and then to assess any wetness. If the leakage is stained blue it is from the bladder, if clear this suggests an ectopic ureter (Freedman and Rickwood 1994). Boys are never continuously wet as a result of an ectopic ureter, but may present later with epididymitis. With any duplication, any portion of the kidney can be smaller, although function is often within normal limits. Reflux into either of the ureters is a potential problem, therefore there is a potential for renal scarring and persistent infections, poor function and ureteric dilation are indications for surgery. Surgery may include a reimplantation of ureters, uretero-ureterostomy, partial nephro-ureterectomy or possibly a heminephro-ureterectomy (Whitaker and Williams 1997).

Nursing issues

Parental anxiety is likely to be greatest when removal of some or all of the kidney is necessary.

It is uncommon to find a wound drain used, but occasionally this may be necessary. Urine output should be monitored initially post-operatively until the child is passing urine well.

Reimplantation of ureters involves a crossing and repositioning of the ureters from the original ureteric orifices. The child may have ureteric stents in place following surgery to aid the healing process. If only one side is affected it is important that urine is passed urethrally following surgery and urinary retention avoided post-anaesthetic. Analgesia is recommended prior to the removal of any drains or stents to minimize significant trauma. Removal of stents is often several days following surgery.

Horseshoe kidney

This is the congenital fusion of the two kidneys into the shape of a horseshoe. The incidence can vary from 1 in 400 to 1 in 1000 (Atwell 1997). It is more common in boys than in girls, and also in approximately one fifth of those affected there are other congenital abnormalities. The horseshoe kidney may also pre-empt obstruction and hydronephrosis.

Ureterocele

This is a cystic dilation of the distal ureter at its insertion (normal or ectopic) into the bladder (Cullinane 1997). The appearance is that of a thin-walled, often translucent mass with the outer surface being vesical epithelium and the inner urethral epithelium, with a thin layer of muscle and collagen between them. Ureteroceles may involve either a single collecting system or the ureter to the upper pole of a duplex system. A ureterocele that is entirely contained within the bladder is usually small and associated with a single collecting system. However, an ectopic ureterocele extends into the bladder neck or urethra and tends to be bigger. It can be disconcerting for a parent to see a ureterocele when changing a nappy and it may have taken them some time to convince others of their sightings. Ureteroceles are not inevitably obstructive; however, there are instances of associated hydronephrosis and hydroureter.

Surgical management to reimplant the ureter and excise the ureterocele may be necessary, depending on the severity of symptoms and any associated obstruction.

Bladder diverticulum

This is a herniation of a pocket of mucosa through a defect in the bladder wall; it may be congenital or acquired. If acquired, a bladder diverticulum is secondary to an obstruction, such as posterior urethral valves or neuropathic bladder. If congenital, then it is more likely in males and due to a developmental defect in the detrusor musculature. Ultimate treatment is excision of the diverticulum with repair of the muscular defect, often via the intravesical route.

Bladder exstrophy (ectopic vesicae)

The incidence of this abnormality has been suggested as 1 in 40 000 live births, and is more common in males than females (Thomas and Barker 1997). The exstrophy is the result of a failure or incomplete closure of the lower anterior abdominal wall due to the ectoderm and endoderm remaining in contact during embryonic development. The absence of intervening mesoderm predisposes to the pelvic viscera becoming laid open on the abdominal surface, with the resultant musculature being normal on each side of the midline defect (Rickwood 1997). In boys, bladder exstrophy is characterized by an absent anterior bladder wall, the pelvic bones are separated and mucosa of the posterior bladder wall bulges outwards due to the raised intra-abdominal pressure. The external sphincter complex is characterized by a fibrous intrapubic bar and is non-functional, the penis is epispadiac (opening on the dorsal side of the penis close to the abdominal wall) and short with an upward chordee, and the prostate and testes are usually normal (Ransley et al. 1989). In females, the anomalies are similar, with a bifida clitoris, abnormal anterior urethral opening, separate vaginal opening and the anus displaced anteriorly. The vagina is often short and the uterus often atypical, with potentially abnormal fertility.

Although it is possible to detect this abnormality antenatally, this is not always the case. Parental anxiety is evident when the baby is born with a clearly visible abnormality. Treatment will mean that the baby is taken to a specialist neonatal surgical centre soon after delivery.

This is a very anxious time for the family as the baby will need corrective surgery within the first few days of life. The immediate concern is to protect the bladder; this is best achieved by covering the bladder with Gelonet. However, clingfilm has been utilized very effectively in practice.

Closure of the bladder is undertaken early, sometimes with the need for pelvic osteotomy, leaving the epispadiac opening for later correction. Bladder drainage following surgery is frequently via a suprapubic catheter left in place for 3–6 weeks, with the pelvic repair being maintained for a similar period by Bryant's traction, hip spica or firm crepe bandage (Rickwood 1997). Vesicoureteric reflux is common following bladder closure, and therefore close management and antibiotic prophylaxis are common. In boys, the epispadias is repaired about age 2–3 years, along with any upward chordee.

The likelihood of attaining 'normal' continence later in life is relatively small (Rickwood 1997). However, reconstructive surgery later in childhood has the potential to offer good urinary control to those who do not attain continence following initial surgery. Bladder augmentation and the formation of a mitrofanoff stoma are approaches that have become popular in recent years. The bladder augmentation acts as a reservoir for urine, with the mitrofanoff being a continent catheterizable channel through which a catheter is passed to drain urine from the bladder, thus promoting continence. For some girls then, urethral catheterization coupled with a bladder neck repair and augmentation can be very effective. However, management of continence is more likely to be different from peers and the urology team need to be mindful not to be overoptimistic at the outset. It should be emphasized that the surgery involved is complex and there is no guarantee of a successful short- or long-term outcome, with the option that a permanent urinary diversion may become the long-term solution of choice (Rickwood 1997).

Nursing issues

During the neonatal period the family will experience considerable stress and anxiety. Fear of holding the baby and undertaking normal baby care may be experienced and reassurance needs to be given. Covering the bladder until such time as closure is possible is imperative; Gelonet or clingfilm can be used. Preservation of the bladder's integrity is important to minimize the infection risk. Once surgery has been carried out the baby is likely to have the mobility of his or her legs restricted to aid healing of the wound and pelvis. The first few days are stressful, as both the urology team and family wait to assess if the initial repair will remain closed. Drainage to the bladder is via a suprapubic catheter that can be left in place for up to 6 weeks. It is not uncommon for the baby to go back to theatre for a second closure, further heightening parental anxiety. Once the wound is healing and the baby is passing urine well, then discharge is arranged, with regular follow-up. Further surgery is likely and this will be planned in stages to maximize on the child's growth and development.

Parental anxieties exist throughout the child's development; frequent hospital outpatient appointments and assessment of renal function will be part of childhood. For boys, anxieties exist relating to sexual development and future sexual relationships. The typical exstrophy penis is short and broad with some degree of erectile deformity (Woodhouse 1989). During adolescence this may become problematic and concern should be given towards helping boys to adjust to their physical appearance. Psychosexual counselling can be helpful as there is no suggestion that libido is altered due to exstrophy for either boys or girls. An optimistic yet realistic view of paternity should be followed, highlighting that until this stage of development is reached it will be difficult to give any concrete answers. Families will need support during this time, especially those families from ethnic cultures. They may find this issue difficult to express, but also have additional anxieties regarding arranged marriages or, where the eldest son was born with exstrophy, sociocultural worries. Cultural anxieties must be recognized, but it is to be hoped that early trusting relationships will enable such issues to be covered and the appropriate support made available for the child and family.

Epispadias

This is a urethral defect where the urethral opening is misplaced dorsally; it can occur anywhere from the glans penis up to the bladder neck.

In the more severe cases, the sphincteric mechanism is almost always affected and continent urinary reconstruction may prove unsuccessful. Reconstruction often begins around the age of 18 months and often involves surgical and postoperative management in line with hypospadias repairs.

For those with poor urinary control, later reconstruction can prove fruitful with the mitrofanoff procedure or possibly an artificial sphincter mechanism.

Labial adhesions

This is a congenital abnormality that occurs when there is a fusion of the labia minora across the midline, obscuring the vaginal orifice. This can be noted soon after birth but may not be recognized until symptoms such as dysuria, dampness or diversion of urinary stream are noted at potty training. Although it is easily rectified it may initially cause some distress to parents and reassurance needs to be given. Topical steroid cream can be applied or the adhesions separated under a general anaesthetic.

Nursing issues

The child, if potty trained, may complain of discomfort when passing urine. Diversional therapy or a warm bath may relieve symptoms. Parents need to be informed that recurrence of adhesions is a possibility.

Urogenital sinus, imperforate anus and cloacal malformation

Although neonates born with congenital abnormalities of the anus, rectum and urogenital sinus are seen initially by a paediatric surgeon, a urologist will have significant input at some stage of reconstruction. Imperforate anus is not uncommon and is usually categorized into four major groups. When the urorectal septum fails to descend completely, a variety of anomalies can be seen, depending on the site of arrested development. Early delay in development in the female will present as persistent cloaca, with the urinary, genital and intestinal tracts meeting in a common channel with a single perineal opening. A communication between the prostatic urethra and the rectum suggests failure of the down growth of the urorectal septum in the male. It is these children who are likely to have urological abnormalities in association with the abnormal presentation of the urogenital openings. With urogenital sinus abnormalities the urethra and the vagina share a common course with a single opening at the vulva.

Stenosis at this point is not uncommon and is associated with hydrometrocolpos and urinary obstruction. This type of abnormality can be seen in females with hypospadias, vaginal atresia and congenital adrenal hyperplasia.

Management commences in the neonatal period and is likely to continue through to early or mid-childhood, depending on the severity of the abnormality. Treatment is likely to be in a regional centre and formation of a colostomy or initial repair will be at the discretion of the paediatric surgeon. The urologist is likely to be involved initially in assessing renal function, possibly formation of a vesicostomy and later with regard to attaining urinary continence. This may involve reconstructive surgery, bladder augmentation and the commencement of intermittent catheterization or formation of a mitrofanoff stoma for catheterization.

Nursing issues

When a child is born with many abnormalities, there can be untold stress on the family. The neonatal period may involve several trips to theatre. The family may not be able to see an end to the surgery or be able to cope with the fact that correction will take place over a period of months or, in some instances, years. It is these families who may become regular visitors to the surgical unit, needing additional support in the community. Furthermore, the teaching of new skills is likely to become a part of care and the paediatric nurse needs to be mindful not to make excessive expectations of the family. Their hopes of a 'normal' childhood for their baby have been shattered and they will need support and counselling to strengthen their resolve during the forthcoming years. Development of a trusting relationship between practitioners, family and child can only serve to strengthen the channels of communication and involve the child and family in any future decision-making process.

Care of the neonate

Initially, the neonate may have both a vesicostomy and a colostomy. Parents may find managing their baby's care in hospital difficult, at a time of increased stress, with anxieties relating to surgery, outcomes and possibly extra financial burdens. Referral to the appropriate services is vital and utilizing practitioners in the hospital, social workers, nurse specialists and paediatric community nurses is likely to aid transition later from hospital to home.

Common obstructive urological disorders

Posterior urethral valves

Posterior urethral valves (PUV), as suggested, are valves within the posterior urethra and exist in boys alone. The primary pathology is a mucosal obstruction in the posterior urethra, existing from embryonic development, with the prostatic urethra developing around 8 weeks of life from the urogenital sinus. Urethral valves as a disease exist on a scale; the severity of outcome is dependent on the timing of the formation of the obstruction during development. Higher obstructions can lead to babies with renal insufficiency, pulmonary hypoplasia and sepsis. Lower and less obstructive valves can lead to a late diagnosis, with the child presenting with a history of incontinence and urinary tract infection. Posterior urethral valves are the commonest cause of lower urinary tract obstruction in male infants. The incidence is between 1 in 8000 and 1 in 25 000 live births. The early stage of urethral obstruction presents secondary problems with regard to altered bladder function and a deterioration in upper tracts and kidneys. Early diagnosis of PUV should be possible with prenatal ultrasonography and regular monitoring of the fetus during development. The baby can be induced early if changes are mapped on ultrasound. Therefore baby boys with PUV born around the gestation age of 35 weeks are not uncommon sights in neonatal surgical units. With advances in endoscopic equipment, the incidence of neonatal mortality for babies with PUV has fallen over recent years. However, for a baby with PUV, success in preserving the renal function is limited significantly by the degree of renal dysplasia (Mitchell and Close 1996). There are a range of approaches to managing the obstructed urethra. The surgical option of diversion is, at this time, not the option of choice as further complications with an already dysfunctional bladder may result. Early ablation of the valves with endoscopic equipment with or without subsequent insertion of suprapubic, urethra catheter or vesicostomy drainage are one approach to management.

Nursing issues

The paediatric practitioner, as with all urological care, has to have an understanding of the pathophysiology of care to be able to support medical staff. This also enables the practitioner to offer explanation to the family, although antenatal diagnosis is a reality for most families.

Care of the neonate

Surgery is undertaken shortly after birth, therefore many families will need additional support because of the separation from their baby at delivery. Ablation of valves can leave the neonate with a urethral catheter or a temporary vesicostomy. The urethral catheter will be removed at the urologist's discretion, possibly 48 hours after surgery. If a vesicostomy is needed then further surgery may not be undertaken for several months, when the baby will be readmitted for closure of the vesicostomy. However the obstructive valves are managed, these children will require long-term follow-up, with regular ultrasound and blood-level monitoring. The involvement of a nephrologist is also important, as up to one third of boys with PUV have impaired renal function in the long term.

Management of continence for children born with PUV

Only recently has the role of the bladder in the outcome of children with valves been highlighted (Mitchell and Close 1996). Urodynamics may have a significant role to play in the long-term management of some children. Early identification of an unstable bladder is important for both continence and long-term outcome. Difficulty with toilet training may be experienced and should be a sign that is flagged up to the urologist. For those children that demonstrate the ability to hold large volumes of urine at high pressures, coupled with residual urine, then alternative methods of bladder emptying need to be found. This could be in the form of intermittent catheterization to promote regular emptying or the formation of a mitrofanoff stoma for those with significant urethral sensation.

Prune-belly syndrome (Triad syndrome, Eagle–Barrett syndrome)

This is characterized by deficient abdominal wall musculature, urinary tract dilation and cryptorchidism. Incidence is approximately 1 in 30 000–50 000 live births, with more males than females affected. The abnormality is visible at birth, with the abdominal wall thin and wrinkled. Problems with the urinary tract are variable and can consist of renal hypoplasia or dysplasia, ureteric dilation, megacystis and dilation of the prostatic urethra. Renal involvement in children ranges from near-normal kidneys to a severe degree of hypoplasia and dysplasia (characterized by the abnormal development of the renal tissue and the presence of primitive ducts in embryonic mesoderm).

The ureters are dilated, elongated, tortuous and thick-walled; obstruction along the length is not uncommon, with the ureteric orifices often wide and patulous. The bladder is enlarged, thickened and non-trabeculated; functionally it can have a large capacity and low voiding pressures. Each case is unique and a urologist should be involved from the early stages, as surgical techniques may be needed to promote effective bladder emptying at a later stage; a mitrofanoff for example. Ultimately some children will also need renal transplant, which may require formation of a urinary diversion prior to the transplant.

Nursing issues

As with congenital conditions, parental anxiety is heightened. If an early picture can be gained regarding renal function and possible long-term outcome, then the nurse needs to be able to support the family in understanding this new information. Interim surgery may be suggested, with the rationale that poorly draining systems invite infection and a deterioration in overall function. Surgery could involve primary diversion via nephrostomy or ureterostomy. Families will need information, an effective listener, and time to be able to assimilate new knowledge and approaches to caring for their baby. Even changing the baby's nappy may be difficult, as anxiety regarding the appearance of the wrinkled abdomen and any stoma can heighten anxiety. Anxieties may also relate to the future likelihood of paternity for this group of children. It has been suggested that functionally, patients with prune-belly syndrome are able to achieve a normal erection but fail to ejaculate. The absence of prostatic and seminal fluid arrests normal spermatic development, therefore psychological counselling is likely to be an area of care incorporated into long-term management with psychosexual counselling offered later.

Further congenital abnormalities of the urethra

Other outflow obstructive abnormalities are very rare but may include polyps of the posterior urethra, mullerian tract abnormalities, urethra duplication (male or female), megalourethra, Cowper's duct syringocele and Skene's duct cysts (Mouriquand and Thomas 1997).

Vesicouretric reflux

This is the retrograde flow of urine. It can give rise to infection, which in turn can lead to ill health in childhood, renal scarring and later hypertension. Furthermore, it can be associated with congenital renal damage (Thomas 1997).

It is usually detected prenatally, clinically with symptoms of a urinary infection, or as an incidental finding during routine investigations of other abnormalities. Initial diagnostics include an ultrasound and micturating cystourethrogram (MCU). Reflux is then graded between I and V (International Relux Study Committee 1981 measurement now widely accepted):

- Grade I: reflux into a non-dilated distal ureter
- Grade II: reflux to level of kidney (pelvis, calices) no dilatation
- Grade III: mild to moderate dilatation but minimal blunting of calices
- Grade IV: moderate dilatation with a loss of angles of fornices, papillary impressions in calices still visible
- Grade V: gross dilatation and tortuosity; impressions of papillae no longer present.

Reflux can stop spontaneously in a large proportion of children (Dawson and Whitfield 1996). Furthermore, continued reflux is not a condition that is considered in isolation, as dysfunctional voiding has a large role to play in the continuation or development of symptoms later in childhood. Conservative management with prophylactic antibiotics, routine follow-up and prompt urinalysis when unwell are common surveillance methods.

Surgery can be indicated and reimplantation of ureters, cutaneous vesicostomy and, more recently, endoscopic correction of the reflux are still practised as management approaches. The endoscopic injection of Teflon into the submucosa of the ureter has had some success. However, concern regarding the risks of migration of Teflon particles has curtailed universal acceptance of the technique. Alternatives to Teflon have been offered, for example collagen paste, but debate regarding use in clinical practice continues (Thomas 1997; Dawson and Whitfield 1996).

Hydronephrosis

Hydronephrosis is renal pelvic dilation with uniformly dilated calices (with or without cortical thinning) (Maizels et al. 1992). Grading of hydrephrosis exists:

- Grade 0: intact central renal complex, normal renal parenchymal thickness
- Grade 1: slight splitting central renal complex, normal renal parenchymal thickness
- Grade 2: evident splitting, complex confined renal border, normal renal parenchymal thickness
- Grade 3: wider splitting, pelvis dilated outside renal border, uniformly dilated calices, normal renal parenchymal thickness
- Grade 4: further dilation of pelvis and calices, thin renal parenchymal thickness (Maizels et al. 1992).

Hydronephrosis can often be detected with antenatal ultrasound, with the baby requiring follow-up with a urologist post-delivery. The effects of hydronephrosis can be progressive, with cortical atrophy, inflammation and scarring all associated with long-standing disease and secondary infection. Hydronephrosis is secondary to obstruction of the urinary tract and it can be unilateral or bilateral. The congenital reasons for hydronephrosis include malformation of the kidney or ureter, obstruction, stones and tumour.

Pelvic–ureteric junction obstruction

Obstruction of the pelvic–ureteric junction may occur during embryonic development, in childhood or in adulthood. This is the commonest obstructive uropathy of childhood, where the essential defect seems to be an aperistaltic segment of ureter from which the normal musculature is congenitally absent (Dawson and Whitfield (1996). Although hydronephrosis is present with obstruction, it has been suggested that not all children will be diagnosed antenatally, and children will continue to present clinically with the complaint. Therefore fetal ultrasonography has limitations in detecting PUJ obstruction (Rickwood 1992). For those children who present with symptoms, abdominal mass or pain, it is more likely that surgery will be indicated. Surgery will also be indicated for obstructive symptoms, stone formation, recurrent urinary infection or progressive renal impairment (Dawson and Whitfield 1996; Rickwood 1997; Rickwood and Godiwalla 1998). A pyeloplasty is the surgical approach to management; this may include the positioning of a ureteric stent and nephrostomy tube (to facilitate drainage of the kidney during the healing process).

Nursing issues

Care of the nephrostomy tube and ureteric stent postoperatively is important to facilitate drainage of the kidney. The time factor with regard to removal of these may be variable, but on average the stent will be removed on day 7–10, with clamping of the nephrostomy tube. If there is no residual urine 24 hours later and no complaint of pain, this can be removed. However, some centres may undertake a nephrostogram prior to removal of a nephrostomy tube.

Both adequate analgesia and diversional play therapy should be utilized with the removal of tubes or stents, with the paediatric nurse acting as an advocate for the child and family to minimize trauma and discomfort for the child.

Tumours

A Wilms' tumour is a malignant embryonal tumour of the kidney, which may metastasize to the lungs, liver and lymph nodes, and is the most common urinary malignancy in children (Dawson and Whitfield 1996; Quaglia 1996). Detection of an abdominal mass is the most common presentation of a Wilms' tumour, although haematuria is present in about a third of cases. Further renal masses in infancy include neuroblastoma, renal adenoma and lymphoma. Not all are malignant therefore a tissue diagnosis is necessary to discriminate a Wilms' tumour from a benign renal mass, such as mesoblastic nephroma (Squire 1997). Diagnosis can be made using ultrasound, demonstrating a solid lesion of the kidney, or intravenous urography, showing distortion and displacement of the calices on the affected side (Dawson and Whitfield 1996). Unfortunately, Wilms' tumours can be bilateral and this needs to be ruled out with investigations to visualize the other kidney. Treatment involves intensive chemotherapy and surgical removal of the tumour at some stage, with radiotherapy usually being used for metastases.

Nursing issues

The child is likely to be nursed on an oncology unit. Surgery is undertaken, possibly after chemotherapy to shrink the tumour. The surgery will involve a nephrectomy. The needs of children and their families during this time is documented in oncology literature.

Rhabdomyosarcoma

A malignant growth of botryoid type, that can present with urological lower uinary tract symptoms such as haematuria and urinary retention. Depending on the growth and position of the tumour, hydronephrosis may be present. Surgery to remove the tumour may necessitate removal of the bladder. Clearly this has implcations later, in that reconstructive surgery to facilitate continence will be needed. Formation of a urinary pouch coupled with a mitrofanoff can be one such approach to attaining continence and reversing a urinary diversion.

Neuropathic bladder

The most common cause of congenital neuropathic bladder is myelomeningocele, with other causes including sacral agenesis, lumbosacral lipoma and, in association, imperforate anus (Rickwood 1997).

The trauma to the innervation of the detrusor and pelvic floor are characteristically the factors that lead to neuropathic bladder, therefore the level of any lesion is important. The parasympathetic innervation to the detrusor and the somatic innervation of the striated musculature of the pelvic floor are rooted via the second, third and fourth sacral segment, therefore low-level lesions are likely to affect the bladder and sphincteric mechanisms. Many congenital neuropathic bladders exhibit a combination of detrusor hyperreflexia and sphincteric incompetence. Voiding is therefore by detrusor contractions and by raising intra-abdominal pressure. Therefore bladder outflow dysfunction, detrusor non-compliancy and detrusor hyper-reflexia not only elicit storage and voiding problems but are factors in secondary upper urinary tract obstruction. If these problems are identified in the neonatal period following investigations such as imaging studies, urodynamics and ultrasound, a vesicostomy may be performed to preserve upper tracts. For those with incompetent bladder neck then safety is maintained, with any degree of reflux being treated with antibiotic prophylaxis.

The attainment of continence becomes a focal point for many children and families, and solutions are sought depending on the child's abilities and motivation. Approaches may include indwelling urinary catheters for girls, penile appliances for boys and, occasionally, permanent urinary diversion (Rickwood 1997). For children with positive conus reflexes, competent sphincteric mechanisms and residual urine, intermittent catheterization coupled with anticholinergic medication can maintain safety and promote being dry. For those children with small residual volumes, incompetent bladder neck or unsafe bladder, surgical options need to be considered. For girls bladder neck suspension with or without bladder augmentation and intermittent catheterization may achieve continence. For boys the use of an artificial sphincter mechanism with or without augmentation and intermittent catheterization may promote continence.

Nursing issues

Any surgical intervention needs to be discussed with the child and family, as it will mean changes in normal routine, which will continue throughout adult life. Open discussion regarding the success of surgery and any future need for surgery should be discussed, as many of these children will have had many hospital admissions. Preoperative counselling is beneficial and liaison with nurse specialists, schools and the primary healthcare team facilitates support for the child and family.

If the child is to have an augmentation then preoperative work-up will include bowel preparation prior to surgery. Following surgery, gastric emptying and hydration will be needed to maintain electrolyte balance. Analgesia should not be compromised, with the false impression that the level of spinal lesion can affect pain threshold. Sensation and pain perception may be altered but it is unlikely to be to such a degree that no pain or discomfort is experienced by the child. Drainage of the bladder will be via either urethral or suprapubic catheters, and there will be an abdominal drain in place. The abdominal drain is usually removed a few days after surgery. If any difficulties are experienced with drainage of the urinary catheter, due to the build up of mucus in the bladder from the augmented bowel, washouts (water/saline for irrigation) may be needed. The augmented bowel will always produce mucus and some children may need washouts to facilitate good drainage for some time following surgery. Removal of the catheter is usually 2–3 weeks following surgery. Intermittent catheterization is then recommenced, taking time to slowly stretch the augmented bladder. It may be necessary to promote overnight drainage of the bladder until such time as it is able to hold good volumes of urine safely.

If an artificial sphincter has been inserted then activation of the device is 6 weeks following surgery. The child needs to be competent in deflating the cuff prior to discharge and again the bladder slowly stretched if an augmentation has been undertaken.

Chapter 4
The kidney and ureter

David Lynes and David Burns

Trauma

Major renal trauma is not uncommon in emergency departments. Knives or gunshot can cause penetrating injuries/wounds. The more common blunt trauma to the kidney should be suspected when an individual presents with pain, bruising and perhaps haematuria.

The kidney is susceptible to crushing between the ribs and lumbar spine. Injury to the loin, ribs or pelvis, often as a result of road traffic accident, sporting injury or falling, can cause blunt kidney damage. Electric shock or invasive procedures such as biopsy can also cause damage. The close proximity of the kidney to other organs and major blood vessels, such as the aorta and inferior vena cava, mean that trauma may not be confined to the kidney.

Haemorrhage is a major problem with both blunt and penetrating kidney traumas. Following blunt trauma the tough Gerotas fascia may remain intact and confine the blood (renal tamponade). A haematoma forms and pressure is put on the kidney, preventing further haemorrhage. If Gerotas fascia is damaged, or if the renal pedicle is torn, bleeding can continue.

Clearly a patient presenting with renal trauma will be in pain and will probably be anxious and shocked. Prime considerations are the maintenance of cardiovascular status, blood volume and renal function. Once the patient has been stabilized, he or she will require investigations; these may include blood for haemoglobin, urea, electrolytes, creatinine, and group and cross match. An angiogram, ultrasound or X-ray may also be required.

Most renal contusions, lacerations and even shattered kidneys can be managed conservatively (Mansi and Alkhudair 1997). The patient should remain on bed rest, and will require intravenous (IV) fluids, and perhaps a blood transfusion. There will be a risk of paralytic ileus if other organs are involved, and if this is suspected the patient should fast until resumption of normal bowel sounds.

Nursing issues

Nursing responsibilities include monitoring bowel sounds, temperature, pulse, blood pressure and girth measurements. Urine output should be measured hourly via a urethral catheter, and sequential samples kept for comparison of haematuria. If haemorrhage is severe or uncontrolled the patient will be prepared for emergency surgery and will require either repair or nephrectomy.

Long-term follow up is important if renal trauma is managed conservatively. Complications can arise days or years post trauma. For example, secondary haemorrhage can occur 10 days after trauma or surgery. Hypertension can occur for a number of reasons and may be transient. If a renal tamponade develops, the haematoma found sub-Gerotas fascia could harden and compress the kidney, causing ischaemia and secretion of the enzyme renin. Renal artery stenosis or renal infarction can also contribute to the secretion of renin and initiation of the renin–angiotensin pathway.

Other complications include hydronephrosis if there is a problem with urethral drainage. Intravenous urography (IVU) on an outpatient basis may be necessary.

Neoplasms

A wide variety of neoplasms affect the kidney. Malignant tumours include Wilms's tumour (also known as nephroblastoma) and renal cell carcinoma (also known as Grawitz tumour, adenocarcinoma, hypernephroma and clear cell carcinoma). The kidneys can also be affected by metastases from other organs, such as the lungs or breast. Benign tumours include adenomas, hemangioma, and angiomyolipoma. Although kidney tumours are relatively rare, they are one of the most common reasons for kidney surgery. Some tumours are increasing in incidence; for example renal cell carcinoma is increasing at a rate of approximately 2% per year.

Wilms' tumours predominantly affect children. Until recently a child with a Wilms' tumour would have a poor prognosis. Recent advances mean that surgical excision and chemotherapy can dramatically improve 5-year survival rates to 80%. Renal cell carcinoma, arising from tubular epithelial cells, accounts for over 80% of all kidney malignancies. It is more common in men than women, and in people over the age of 50. Symptoms, treatment and prognosis depend largely on the stage of renal cell carcinoma. Staging categories typically start with a small tumour that is confined to the kidney with no invasion of perinephric fat. The other extreme is a tumour that has invaded the abdominal wall, adjacent organs, local and regional lymphatic tissue, with distant metastases to organs such as the brain, lungs and liver.

A person with renal cell carcinoma may be asymptomatic or may present with haematuria (not always present even in advanced disease), pain, weight loss, anaemia, hypertension and erythrocytosis. Invasion of the inferior vena cava may cause bilateral leg oedema.

Investigations for kidney neoplasms include IVU, computerized tomography (CT) scan (for staging), ultrasound, magnetic resonance imaging (MRI), angiography, radionuclide imaging and urine for cytology.

If renal cell carcinoma is confined to the kidney, post-treatment 5-year survival rate can be 80%. Radical nephrectomy is the treatment of choice, with radiotherapy if there is evidence of local invasion. Metastases can be removed surgically if they are small in number. If widespread metastases are evident treatment is palliative. Radiotherapy or embolization may prove effective in the treatment of symptoms. The palliative care team should be involved.

The results of chemotherapy trials have been poor; no regime has significantly reduced renal cell carcinoma. Occasionally, even in the absence of treatment, there have been 'miracle' cures or spontaneous regression of tumours and secondaries. This has prompted research into the role of the body's own immune response to tumour cells and the search for the right stimulus for an immune response. Results of clinical trials with Calmette–Guérin bacillus (BCG) vaccine, interferon and interleukin-2 look promising, and have significantly altered the treatment of metastatic renal cell carcinoma. Trials that combine interleukin-2 and interferon have produced a response rate of 25%, and an average survival rate of more than 3 years (Rosenberg et al. 1989; Atzpodien et al. 1990).

Nursing issues

Factors that the nurse should consider when caring for the patient with renal cell carcinoma include the patient's anxiety about prognosis and fear of losing a kidney. There is a need to provide information and other health education strategies.

Postoperative nephrectomy care includes the care of thoracic and renal drains, with a specific focus on blood loss at the drain site. There is an increased risk of haemorrhage and pulmonary embolus if the inferior vena cava is involved. Urine output via a urethral catheter should be monitored, and should exceed 0.5 ml per kg of body weight per hour. Paralytic ileus can be a potential problem if the small intestine has been handled, and oral fluids should be introduced gradually. Pain control is an important aspect of postoperative care.

Kidney infection

Pyelonephritis is infection and inflammation of the kidney and renal pelvis. It usually occurs when bacteria enter collecting ducts after ascending the ureter(s). Reflux and back pressure of urine can force urine up the collecting ducts. Bacteria can also enter the kidneys via the blood, although this is comparatively rare, and in this case pyelonephritis is described as haematogenous in origin.

The pelvis and renal parenchyma become inflamed, and abscesses and suppuration can develop. The glomeruli are resistant to acute infection but tubules can be destroyed. If treated effectively, kidney infections rarely lead to disease or kidney failure (USDOH 1991). Repeated acute episodes can lead to scarring and nephrosis; the kidney shape becomes irregular, fibrosis occurs and drainage is impaired. Chronic pyelonephritis, involving repeated cycles of scarring, papillary necrosis and deteriorating renal function, develops. Chronic and occasionally acute renal failure can occur, and the patient may become hypertensive due to renal ischaemia. In extreme cases the whole kidney can suppurate. Gerotas fascia in effect becomes a bag of pus, and there is a risk of septicaemia. Pyelonephritis can be life threatening.

Factors that predispose people to kidney infection include lower urinary tract infection and the potential for reflux. Diabetes, immunosuppression and catheterization all increase the risk of infection, whereas calculi, refluxing ureters, neuropathic bladder and prostatic hyperplasia increase the risk of obstruction or stasis.

A person suffering from an acute episode of pyelonephritis will feel ill. He or she will be pyrexial and may be in pain. General malaise, nausea, vomiting and anorexia may all be experienced. The patient may feel discomfort when voiding (dysuria) and the urine may be cloudy with leukocytes (pyuria). Elderly patients may become incontinent and acutely confused.

Nursing issues

Nursing considerations include increasing fluid intake IV and orally, if tolerated, and IV antibiotics. Control of symptoms such as pain, nausea and pyrexia are important to the client. Urine output should be monitored carefully.

Tests the client may undergo include urinalysis, ultrasound, voiding cystourethrography, CT scan, excretion urography and IVU. Pyelonephritis will be evident in the form of obstruction, shrinkage and deformity. If damage is extensive, unilateral and accompanied by hypertension, the patient may need a nephrectomy. Long-term care may include removal of the obstruction and minimizing risk factors. Health education plays a large role. Hygiene should be discussed. Sexually active women should be encouraged to completely empty their bladder after intercourse, thereby flushing out any bacteria forced into the urethra during coitus.

Stones

Urolithiasis, a stone (calculus) in the urinary tract, is recognized as one of the most painful disorders. Stones can occur anywhere in the renal collecting and drainage system. Nephrolithiasis refers to a stone in the kidney, ureterolithiasis in the ureter(s).

The incidence of urolithiasis is increasing annually in the West. Approximately 12% of people will experience renal calculi at some time in their lives, and it is three times more common in men than in women (Hanno and Wein 1994).

Stones can be formed from a number of substances that may be found in urine, for example calcium, oxalate, phosphate and urate. These substances can precipitate, especially if there is an existing nucleus, such as a piece of old stone or dead tissue. A reduction in urine flow due to, for example, obstruction can increase the chances of their development.

Calculi can also be formed from substances not normally present in urine, or present in excessive quantities. Cystine is an amino acid that is normally reabsorbed by the tubule. It will be present in the urine if there is a genetic defect preventing reabsorption. The drug penicillamine helps to make cystine soluble and prevent the formation of stones.

Homeostatic disorders such as hypercalcaemia, either idiopathic or due to hyperparathyroidism, can cause calcium to precipitate. Parathyroidectomy can help in these circumstances. Alteration of the pH of urine can encourage precipitation of substances. Renal tubular acidosis lowers pH and infection can raise pH due to bacteria converting urea into ammonia.

Maintaining an adequate fluid intake can help prevent all types of urolithiasis.

Once formed, stones can obstruct the drainage system. The ureters above the calculi can dilate due to build-up of urine, which is forced into surrounding tissues through extravasation. Peristaltic movements of the urethra attempt to move the stone. The net result is an extremely painful condition called renal colic. Pain can be so extreme that it causes hyperventilation, nausea and vomiting.

The patient presenting with a renal stone may undergo several investigations, which can include urinalysis and culture, renal ultrasound, X-ray, IVU, pyelography, CT scan and radionuclide renography. Most stones will appear on a plain X-ray, though some stones are (rarely) translucent. Plain X-ray will also reveal the presence of ureteric stones either singly or in a line known as the Steinstrasse effect. Causes, including metabolic, should also be ruled out.

Urolithiasis can be treated conservatively. IV or oral fluids encourage most stones to pass spontaneously. Urine should be sieved to check for stones or 'gravel'. In some cases ureteric stenting or lasertripsy is needed. Invasive procedures such as percutaneous nephrolithotomy are now performed infrequently. They are reserved for larger stones or for when other methods have failed. Postoperative considerations include encouraging fluids, and being aware of the danger of infection and haemorrhage.

The treatment of choice for upper renal tract stones is currently extracorporeal lithotripsy, or shock wave therapy. Shock waves are obtained from a spark generator or piezoelectric dish. They are directed at the stones with the help of X-ray or ultrasound. The shock waves require water as a transmission medium and at least part of the patient's body will be in contact with water.

Extracorporeal lithotripsy machines were first used in the early 1980s and have undergone developments since then. Older machines, still in use at many centres, involve the anaesthetized patient being strapped into a chair and lowered into a bath. The patient is catheterized to avoid urine entering the bath water. Complications include bruised skin, pain and the possibility of kidney damage. More modern machines involve the patient lying on a small basin of fluid. The patient is not immersed. The shocks are not severe and the patient requires neither analgesia nor a catheter. Bruising and discomfort are not a problem.

With all extracorporeal lithotripsy the patient may require repeated treatment. Fluids should be encouraged postoperatively and the urine sieved for gravel. The nurse should be alert for signs of sepsis and renal colic.

Upper renal tract drainage problems

Drainage problems can occur due to compression, obstruction or narrowing of the ureters. This in turn can lead to pain, fever, hydronephrosis and uraemia.

Conditions that can result in drainage problems include tuberculosis, bilharziasis (caused by the flatworm *Schistosoma*), stones, changes in the ureter due to chronic renal tract obstruction, cancer, pelvic–ureteric junction obstruction, retroperitoneal fibrosis and congenital abnormalities.

Pelvic–ureteric junction obstruction is caused by an idiopathic ring of fibrous tissue at the point where the renal pelvis becomes narrower and forms the ureter. Back pressure of urine causes the renal pelvis to become stretched and distorted, leading to pain and vomiting. The obstruction can be resolved through surgical alteration of the pelvic–ureteric junction (pyeloplasty). This involves using surplus renal pelvis to widen the narrowed portion of the ureter. The anastomosis may need to be supported by a splinting catheter for several days. This should be clamped prior to removal, and any signs of fever or discomfort indicate problems with the patency of the ureter.

Retroperitoneal fibrosis involves the formation of fibrous tissue behind the peritoneum. The condition is more common in men than women. The ureters become compressed and distorted, and drainage is restricted. Steroids can slow the progression of retroperitoneal fibrosis. Surgical intervention involves freeing the ureters from fibrous tissue, and wrapping them in omentum thereby avoiding the risk of further involvement with fibrous tissue.

Stenosis and obstruction of the ureters can be relieved by surgical intervention, dilatation, ureteral stenting or percutaneous nephrostomy.

Dilation of the ureter is often attempted for non-malignant ureteral strictures. It can avoid the use of a chronic indwelling stent, although a temporary stent may be required post-dilatation in order to maintain the patency of the ureter while the muscles heal.

Stents can be used to decompress the ureter, for example when a secondary tumour is involved. They can be inserted and replaced using a cystoscope, or when retrograde insertion is difficult percutaneous stenting is possible.

Percutaneous nephrostomy involves the insertion of a silicone tube into the renal pelvis under local anaesthetic. Clients often see this as less convenient and comfortable due to the surgical incision and a sutured 'plate', which holds the tube in place.

Vascular disorders

The kidneys receive 25% of the blood supply with each heartbeat and, as outlined in Chapter 1, have a crucial role in maintaining blood pressure. This ability to deliver large amounts of blood to the kidneys is essential for their normal functioning. It is unsurprising therefore that disturbance of blood supply will result in a failure to maintain at least one, but usually more, aspects of homeostasis.

In terms of disturbed blood supply, Long and Phipps (1995) described three major types of vascular disorder:

• renal artery stenosis
• nephrosclerosis
• diabetic nephropathy.

Renal artery stenosis involves a narrowing of the renal artery, usually as a result of atheromatous plaques, which may be caused by factors such as a fatty diet and smoking. Thrombosis and emboli can also contribute to the partial or complete occlusion of the renal artery. In women, a further cause of stenosis is recognized, fibromuscular dysplasia. Here there is a picture of alternating narrowing and dilatation of the renal artery, giving what Gauntlett-Beare and Myers (1994) describe as a 'necklace' picture on angiogram.

Whereas renal artery stenosis is confined to the major renal artery, nephrosclerosis is a more diffuse phenomenon. It affects the microvascular structures within the kidneys. Nephrosclerosis is often caused by hypertension and develops gradually, although in patients who develop acute and severe hypertension, renal failure can occur almost immediately. In the less acute form of nephrosclerosis, renal arterioles have thickened and narrowed lumens. These changes extend to the glomerular capillaries and the renal tubules. Nephrosclerosis is a major cause of chronic renal failure.

Willis (1995b) states that over 25% of people with diabetes are likely to develop diabetic nephropathy, and that this condition is the most common reason for long-term dialysis in the UK. Pathophysiological changes include thickening of the capillary basement membrane in the glomerulus, a fall in glomerular filtration rate (GFR) and a gradually increasing proteinuria. The Diabetes Control and Complications Group (1993) has been hailed as a landmark in the management of diabetic patients. This trial demonstrated conclusively that good diabetic control dramatically reduces the incidence and progression of diabetic nephropathy and other diabetes-related complications.

Of the three categories of vascular disorders described, only renal artery stenosis is amenable to surgical intervention such as angioplasty. Even in this instance, surgery is not always possible because the atheromatous plaques do not usually exist in isolation. The main causes of vascular problems in the kidney are more amenable to appropriate health education in relation to diet, smoking and exercise.

Renal failure

Renal failure is the inability to maintain fluid and electrolyte balance, to excrete waste products and to control blood pressure. Some authors have defined renal failure as a daily urine output of less than 400 ml; however, this is a generalization and diagnosis is made on an individual basis. Renal failure can be classified as acute or chronic.

Acute renal failure

Conventionally, acute renal failure has been divided into three types: pre-renal, intra-renal and post-renal acute renal failure.

Pre-renal acute renal failure occurs when there is a loss of pressure in the renal artery. Common causes include hypovolaemia (due to dehydration, burns, haemorrhage), vasodilation (anaphylaxis, septicaemia) or 'pump' failure, as occurs in cardiogenic shock. The kidney structure is unaltered and the potential for adequate renal function remains, but the kidneys are underperfused with blood. The monitoring of blood pressure and restoration of adequate blood supply to the kidneys is essential if damage to the proximal convoluted tubules is to be avoided.

Intra-renal acute renal failure involves the basic functional unit of the kidney, the nephron. Antigen/antibody complexes may block these, for example following streptococcal infections, subacute bacterial endocarditis or polyarteritis nodosa. The nephron may also be deprived of blood due to pre-renal acute renal failure, and will develop impairment of function due to hypoxia and tubule damage. Toxic substances can damage the nephron. These include heavy metals such as mercury or gold, antibiotics such as gentomycin or tetracycline, analgesics such as paracetamol or ibuprofen, or cytotoxic substances such as methotrexate or bleomycin.

Post-renal acute renal failure occurs when an obstruction distal to the nephron prevents the formation of new urine. Examples include renal calculi and neoplasms.

Nursing issues

One of the most crucial elements of the nurse's role is monitoring fluid intake and output, and recording the patient's weight each day. Only 500 ml of fluid plus the previous day's urinary output is given. The 500 ml accounts for the 'insensible' loss, i.e. water lost through the skin, lungs and bowels. By adding the previous day's urinary output to this volume the kidneys are given as much 'work' as they have demonstrated they can handle. Any fluid intake in excess of this calculated figure can lead to fluid overload and cardiac failure.

Accurate fluid recording is, therefore, essen[t]
patient with his or her maximum fluid intake
avoiding fluid overload. Unfortunately there
balance recording is not as accurate as it c[o]
found major discrepancies between various g
of the volumes they ascribed to four commonl[y]
Finlay (1989) refers to the notoriously inaccurate fluid balance chart.

Complementary to fluid recording is the recording of the patient's weight. Many practitioners find this more reliable, as trends in water gain and loss are more easily discernible. To ensure accuracy, the patient should be weighed on the same scales, at the same time of day, in similar clothes, every day. It may also be advisable to weigh the patient without checking the previous day's weight as this may lead to some bias on the observer's part.

Diet is another important nursing consideration. The liver converts excess protein into energy and urea by a process of deamination. Protein restriction can slow down the rise in uraemia. Garrett (1995) reviews the nutritional management of acute renal failure and makes several points, including the fact that the mortality of acute renal failure has not improved greatly despite modern antibiotics and careful dietary controls, although the latter is still debatable among clinicians. Garrett indicates that severe protein restriction may be harmful as it can lead to muscle wasting and infection. Ideally, protein intake needs to be geared towards the individual's needs. Modest protein restriction will help control rises in urea, but for severely ill patients with increased metabolic rates, protein intakes may have to be increased in order to maintain lean body mass. A high carbohydrate diet is protein-sparing and excess urea can be removed by dialysis.

The kidney has a major function in maintaining optimum levels of serum electrolytes and an electrolyte imbalance is inevitable with acute renal failure. There is a particular risk of sodium and potassium retention. Sodium is important for the maintenance of extracellular fluid volume. If potassium levels rise (hyperkalcaemia), cardiac arrhythmias can become life threatening. A low sodium and potassium diet may be required. Potassium levels can also be reduced by the intravenous administration of glucose and insulin, as potassium enters body cells with glucose.

High levels of urea predispose to bleeding and infection, and the nurse should be alert to the development of these problems.

ıc renal failure

pproximately 3500 people present with end stage renal failure
(ESRF) in the UK each year. Half of these have either chronic
glomerulonephritis or chronic pyelonephritis. Other causes include
diseases of the vasculature, for example secondary to diabetes or
hypertension; polycystic kidneys; and hereditary or congenital factors.

In contrast to patients with acute renal failure, patients with
chronic renal failure usually experience polyuria because of the
kidneys' inability to concentrate urine. Patients may retain sodium
and develop acidosis. Calcium absorption may be poor due to failure
to synthesize 1,25-dihydroxycholecalciferol, which can lead to osteomalacia. Urea and creatinine rise and the patient develops anaemia.
Various other problems such as gout, pericarditis and bleeding can
develop due to inability to remove toxins.

The management of chronic renal failure is aimed at slowing the
progression of, and compensating for, failing renal function. Vitamin
D in high doses is given for osteomalacia. Hypertension is managed
with appropriate drugs and health education. Blood transfusions
may be required for anaemia. Diet is again an important consideration. It is likely that protein will be restricted to control uraemia. The
patient may need a high or low sodium diet, and a low potassium
diet, depending on blood electrolyte measurements. A low protein,
low salt diet is unpleasant to eat and it is important to liaise with the
dietician to discuss palatable options.

Fluid intake should be modified to meet the patient's requirements. If the patient is passing large volumes of urine, adequate
intake is needed to avoid dehydration. If urine output is low, fluid
intake is reduced and the patient weighed each day to check for fluid
retention.

Uraemia can cause the patient several problems. The pigment of
the skin alters and the skin may become itchy. There is an increased
risk of bleeding, infection and pericarditis. The patient will be tired,
breathless and generally unwell if he or she is anaemic. Men may
develop gynaecomastia and may become impotent. Altered body
image is an important consideration when nursing the patient with
chronic renal failure.

If conservative treatment fails, patients will need to move on to
some form of dialysis.

Dialysis

Renal dialysis uses the processes of osmosis and diffusion to modify the plasma concentration of water and various other substances. If a semi-permeable membrane separates two solutions of unequal compositions, the substances in the solution will cross the membrane and both solutions will eventually become identical in composition. Substances such as sodium, urea and potassium move across the membrane by diffusion; water crosses the membrane by osmosis. Pressure can also be used to force water across a membrane in some circumstances. It is possible to alter the composition of blood by placing it and a prepared fluid – the dialysate – in contact with opposite sides of a semi-permeable membrane. In this way, water and various other substances can be added to and removed from the blood.

There are two major types of dialysis, peritoneal dialysis and haemodialysis. Peritoneal dialysis uses the patient's peritoneum, the thin cellular membrane that covers the abdominal organs. This membrane is supplied with a blood capillary network. Dialysate is instilled into the peritoneal cavity for a period of time, and then removed. Peritoneal dialysis has the advantage that it may be undertaken while the patient carries on with their normal, everyday routine. In this case it is referred to as continuous (or chronic) ambulatory peritoneal dialysis (CAPD).

Haemodialysis involves an extracorporeal dialysing machine, which takes blood from the patient, passes it through a dialysis mechanism and subsequently returns it to the patient. The dialysis mechanism contains a manmade semi-permeable membrane. As blood is transported to and from a dialysis machine during haemodialysis, reliable access to the cardiovascular system is required. This usually involves the radial artery and cephalic vein, and a surgically developed arteriovenous fistula. The fistula causes the vein to become thickened and distended, thereby enabling easier access.

Nursing issues

The nursing care of a patient undergoing haemodialysis is complex, and a comprehensive review is beyond the scope of this chapter. Factors that should be taken into consideration include health education and preparation of the patient, who has a large part to play in ensuring the success of dialysis. The periods of time between dialysis are crucial. During these times various substances cannot be removed from the plasma because the patient's kidney function is severely impaired. There is the potential for their rapid accumulation. Potassium intake should be restricted to minimize the risk of hyperkalcaemia. A low sodium diet is important because the accumulation of sodium can lead to pulmonary and systemic oedema, hypertension and heart failure. Fluid intake should be carefully controlled. The patient will also require vitamin and iron supplements to compensate for loss during dialysis.

Chapter 5
The bladder

PHILIP DOWNEY

Bladder dysfunction

Detrusor dysfunction

Paralysis of the bladder can follow surgical intervention where pelvic parasympathetic pathways are cut or removed (such as radical hysterectomy). It can also occur after sustaining a pelvic fracture if the nerves are torn during the accident. The bladder is then demonstrated in urodynamics as being big and floppy, with no detrusor contractions. The somatic nerves may be intact and the sphincter may also obstruct outflow from the bladder.

Predisposing conditions, such as diabetes, may also give rise to one of two clinical pictures. The bladder could appear to be hypersensitive, and may empty when less than completely full and yet not completely empty itself on voiding.

Alternatively, the appearance may be of an overdistended bladder with a large residual volume. Urodynamic studies would indicate weak detrusor contractions, large residual volume and a relative obstruction of the bladder neck (Blandy 1991). This is commonly labelled as detrusor instability.

Treatment of detrusor instability

Initially, the patient (if being treated as an inpatient) may be catheterized using a urethral or suprapubic catheter. The patient will then commence oral medication in the form of alpha blockers, such as

Tamsulosin or Indoramin, which will relax smooth muscle. This will be followed 48 hours later by a trial without catheter.

The patient will then be expected to perform a flow rate and a residual ultrasound scan would be appropriate. If necessary, the patient will be taught how to perform clean intermittent self-catheterization (CISC).

If the individual is attending for urodynamics as an outpatient, the use of alpha blockers (without catheterization) may be appropriate. The patient should then be asked to record a 'time and amount chart' ready for their next outpatient review, in an attempt to observe any improvement in amounts being voided.

In cases where the patient complains of frequency – passing little urine but very often – treatment of the irritable detrusor may be required. In cases such as this, antimuscarinic drugs such as oxybutynin 2.5 mg (increasing to 5 mg) orally may well be acceptable in calming down the bladder. This type of drug helps to increase bladder capacity by reducing the unstable detrusor contractions. At present, there is no licensed intravesical drug therapy for detrusor irritation, but experience in Liverpool shows that instillation of oxybutynin into the bladder is a very effective method of treating detrusor irritability.

Bladder outflow obstruction

This is common in men with an enlarged prostate or urethral stricture. With increased outflow obstruction, the detrusor responds by becoming stronger. Initially, the wall of the bladder will become thickened. At first, the increased power of the detrusor keeps the bladder empty, and the flow rate appears to be maintained. There may be some frequency and urgency at this stage. The stream may appear to be unaffected. After a while, the detrusor will weaken and the bladder no longer empties itself. As a result, the residual volume of urine grows and become a potential focus for infection.

As time passes, the residual volume will become so large that the individual can suffer with chronic retention. The bladder wall by this stage tends to be fibrous tissue. The ureter will become dilated with hydronephrosis due to back pressure, and renal failure becomes a reality.

Retention of urine

This is classed as a medical emergency. The patient needs to be catheterized – preferably urethrally (because of unknown bladder pathology). If the patient is severely strictured or has a profoundly enlarged prostate, he or she could be catheterized using a suprapubic catheter.

Acute retention of urine

This is retention of rapid onset, and can occur not only in prostate disease or urethral strictures, but can happen spontaneously in post-operative cases or in situations of severe constipation.

Treatment is by catheterization, followed by a trial without catheter after 48 to 72 hours. If the patient is constipated, this needs treatment with aperients and/or laxatives prior to the trial without catheter.

During the trial without catheter, the patient should perform a flow rate and also have a residual volume ultrasound scan performed. If the patient is unable to void, and complains of lower abdominal pains, the medical staff should be informed. The patient will then need to be recatheterized, with an alternative treatment plan decided upon.

Chronic retention of urine

This is retention that occurs over a period of time. Usually the patient is unaware of the problem until they are suddenly unable to void. They may have experienced a slower and weaker stream on micturition, but ignored this as either a sign of ageing, or other such cause. As with acute retention, the treatment is classed as a medical emergency and the individual will require catheterization.

Nursing observations include monitoring urinary output. While monitoring output, the nurse will notice a large diuresis, e.g. 2 litres within two hours of catheterization. Common practice among nurses used to be to clamp the catheter to prevent the patient going into shock. However, it needs to be noted, that A CATHETER SHOULD NEVER BE CLAMPED, because a clamp can be forgotten.

If such a diuresis is recorded it needs to be reported to medical staff. The large diuresis occurs due to the catheterization – much in the same way as releasing a plug from a bath! When the catheter is inserted, the plug is released. However, in chronic retention, the kidneys are used to having to excrete urine under considerable pressure due to hydronephrosis. Once the pressure drops, the kidneys continue to diurese at the increased pressure, thereby producing a greater volume of urine than normal. In this state, the kidneys are described as decompressing.

Treatment for the large diuresis centres around exactly how much urine is being produced. Hourly measurements are essential. This fluid output needs to be replaced in a fluid chase; i.e. previous hour's output = next hour's intravenous (IV) input.

Serum urea and electrolytes need to be monitored on a regular basis in an attempt to prevent the patient dehydrating. After 48–72 hours, provided the urea and electrolytes remain stable, the fluid chase can be stopped and replaced with an IV regimen of 3 litres/24 hours. Subsequent treatment of the cause of chronic retention can then be decided upon.

Bladder cancer

This is a very common urological malignancy, which presents in various stages and varieties. Globally, it is seen as being common mainly within the industrialized nations and especially in people who have worked in the rubber industry or those working with certain chemicals. Smoking is also another contributory factor.

Classification of the disease is made using an internationally agreed staging system, i.e. the TNM (tumour, nodes and metasteses) and G (Gleason) stages (Table 5.1).

Table 5.1 Bladder tumour staging

Stage	Meaning
T 1	Superficial tumour confined to bladder mucosa
T 2	Invasion of superficial muscle
T 3	Invasion of deep muscle
T 4	Tumour invading other organs/tissues

Patients with some forms of bladder cancer tend to present with one or more episodes of painless haematuria (Fenwick 1997). The haematuria, while painless, may also be microscopic and only diagnosed by urinary dipstick (routine urinalysis).

Other individuals will not experience haematuria, but may instead present with pyuria, which fails to grow anything on microscopic culture.

People presenting with any of these symptoms will benefit from renal ultrasound scans and flexible cystoscopy, as well as a routine serum urea and electrolyte profile in an attempt to allow diagnosis.

Transurethral resection of bladder tumour

Treatment options for bladder cancer are numerous, and will depend on the staging and diagnosis of the disease (Table 5.2). All patients will require a cystoscopy under general anaesthetic, and subsequent histology of the biopsies obtained from the initial transurethral resection of tumour (known as TURT or TURBT).

Table 5.2 Bladder tumour treatment options

Stage	Options
T 1	Intravesical chemotherapy
	Laser therapy/traditional TURT
T 2	TURT with or without radiotherapy or chemotherapy
	Cystodiathermy
	Possible cystectomy
T 3	Radiotherapy/chemotherapy
	Ileal conduit formation
	Possible continent diversion following partial cystectomy
T 4	Palliative symptom control
	Nephrostomies +/− ureteric stenting

Nursing care post-TURT

This will include care of the bladder irrigation and maintaining hydration through an IV infusion until the patient is able to eat and drink. Vital signs need to be recorded on a regular basis due to the possibility of haemorrhage and hypovolaemic shock.

The saline irrigation can be discontinued when the amount of haematuria subsides, and the catheter removed as indicated by the medical staff. This should be done preferably at midnight on the day of choice (Downey et al. 1997).

TUR syndrome

Perioperatively, glycine bladder irrigation is used in cystoscopic resection due to non-conductive properties when using the diathermy.

As with all surgery involving glycine bladder irrigation in theatre, there is a real possibility of the patient experiencing TUR syndrome. The nurse needs to be vigilant for this – observing for a rise in blood pressure and for reduced urinary output; on occasions, the patient will complain of flashing lights in their eyes or even blindness.

TUR syndrome occurs due to the absorption of the glycine in theatre. It is treated by monitoring serum urea and electrolytes (usually sodium will fall) and the administration of IV saline 0.9%. Natural reaction for the inexperienced nurse or junior doctor would be to give IV frusemide because it appears that the patient is over-loaded. Discussion surrounds the value of this (Steggall 1999). However, most experienced staff decide not to give frusemide, because it appears to worsen the effects, and lower the serum sodium even further.

Laser TURT

This produces very little bleeding, and in many cases there is no need for urethral catheterization. As a result, individuals undergoing laser TURT will be classed as day-case patients who attend for a general anaesthetic routine check cystoscopy.

Individuals undergoing laser TURT appear to have the same tumour recurrence rate as conventional TURT patients (Fenwick 1997).

Nursing care post-laser TURT

Nursing care is minimal. Urinary output should be recorded to ensure that the patient has voided. Vital signs should be monitored also.

Photodynamic therapy

This is used when an individual has a superficial but solid tumour of the bladder. This treatment involves injecting a photosensitizer and destroying the tumour with laser beams of a certain frequency (Fenwick 1997).

The patient is given the photosensitizer by IV injection, which is then taken up by the normal and tumour cells. Cancer cells will retain the drug and the normal cells will excrete the agent. The patient then attends theatre and receives the laser under direct visual control.

Nursing care postoperatively

The patient needs to be observed for urinary output and voiding patterns. They will commonly experience frequency and suprapubic pains, often requiring analgesia.

On discharge home, the patient should be advised to stay out of sunlight for 2–3 weeks, due to the rate of metabolizing the photosensitive agent.

Irritation can be experienced for up to 3 months, along with sloughing of tissue. Haematuria may also appear during this period and advice regarding this possibility should be explained.

Superficial bladder tumours

Intravesical chemotherapy

Intravesical chemotherapy is generally used for superficial cancers, and can be done as a day case. During this procedure, the bladder mucosa is exposed to a chemotherapy agent, killing as many malignant cells as possible, but also reducing the risk of damaging the normal healthy mucosa (Fenwick 1997).

The patient is catheterized using a catheter without a balloon, such as a Nelaton catheter. The solution is then passed into the bladder through this catheter, which is subsequently removed and disposed of after instilling the solution.

Individuals undergoing this procedure are then asked to retain the solution, turning from the supine position to one side after 15 minutes, then on to their abdomen after another 15 minutes, and finally on to their other side for the last 15 minutes, taking one hour in total to coat the surface of the bladder. The patient should then be advised to void directly into a toilet in order to prevent contamination of other people.

Common solutions used in intravesical chemotherapy include mitomycin and BCG (Calmette-Guérin bacillus). Individuals may complain of side effects from this type of treatment (e.g. experiences of flushing sensations, etc.). These should be observed and recorded, and where necessary reported as an adverse drug reaction if they are not recognized symptoms.

Stage II bladder tumours

These are more invasive than superficial tumours, and their management involves methods which can penetrate beyond the superficial bladder mucosa.

The treatment of choice for this type of tumour includes TURT in combination with either chemotherapy or radiotherapy. Decisions surrounding the choice between chemotherapy or radiotherapy will be made following the histological report.

Follow-up check cystoscopies should be carried out for a 10-year period to ensure that regrowth has not occurred.

Stage III bladder tumours

These are more serious than the others with regard to the patient's prognosis. These tumours will have deeply invaded the muscle of the bladder wall, and if left without treatment will spread beyond the bladder.

The urologist may decide to refer the patient for radiotherapy prior to surgery, although this may cause problems with wound healing and bladder wall adhesion when the time to operate arrives. Usually, the surgeon will operate first.

In virtually all cases, the treatment of choice will be to perform either an ileal conduit formation plus or minus total cystectomy and possible urethrectomy.

Preparation of the patient for ileal conduit formation

This will be a traumatic time for the patient and his or her partner. The operation will involve the resection of a piece of ileum, which is brought to the surface of the abdominal wall to form a stoma. The ureters are then resected and implanted into the stoma.

Due to the formation of a stoma, referral to a stoma nurse is appropriate, in order that the patient and their partner can have preoperative counselling and the right to choose an appropriate appliance. Part of the stoma nurse's role is to mark the site of the stoma for the surgeon. This is done after a discussion with the patient, where lifestyle and hobbies are taken into account. Body image changes are inevitable, and the role of the stoma nurse cannot be ignored.

Physical preparation will include some form of bowel preparation. The patient will be advised to take a fluids only diet for 48 hours preoperatively. Discussion surrounds the use of aperients for this type of surgery. Latest research shows that patients recover at a faster rate with minimal disturbance in serum urea and electrolytes if no aperient is used – and there is only the administration of a mini-enema on the night prior to surgery (Downey and Fordham 1998).

Nursing care post-ileal conduit formation

Vital signs need to be recorded at regular intervals postoperatively. The patient will return to the ward with an analgesic device such as an epidural or patient-controlled analgesia (PCA) pump. They will have an IV infusion in progress until they are able to eat and drink (between 5 to 10 days on average depending upon bowel sounds).

The stoma should be pink and healthy, with two ureteric stents draining into the stoma bag. (These stents are usually removed after 10 days.) Initially, for the first two days, the output should be recorded hourly, with a preferred rate of 50 ml/hr being the accepted drainage.

There will be an abdominal wound, which should be checked on a regular basis and redressed when indicated. Usually the patient will have wound drains. These need close observation, and will be removed once the ureteric stents have removed at day 10.

Until the patient is fully mobile, he or she should wear anti-embolic stockings and receive subcutaneous injections of heparin. When the patient is fully mobile, drains and sutures have been removed, and he or she is able to perform a bag change with the stoma nurse, the patient will be discharged home.

In men undergoing this type of radical surgery there will be a virtual 100% chance of impotence due to the disruption of nerve pathways (Fenwick 1997).

Stage IV bladder tumours

This stage involves the invasion of the tumour through the bladder wall and into surrounding structures. They are, in all reality, beyond extensive surgical treatment, and are within the remit of palliative care.

Treatment options include temporary urinary diversion, nephrostomy tube insertion (with antegrade ureteric stenting where possible), strong analgesia, radiotherapy and psychological care.

Incontinence of urine

Over recent years there has been an attempt to regulate the terminology associated with urinary incontinence (ICS 1984). It can take a variety of forms, and these include:

- Stress incontinence: this occurs when there is a failure of the urethral sphincter to remain closed when a sudden increase in abdominal pressure occurs (during sneezing or coughing for example). The pelvic floor is weak and allows the urethra to descend and the sphincter to open, thus allowing urine to leak.
- Urge incontinence: this results from the contraction of the detrusor muscle as though the person is to void when there is only a small volume of urine in the bladder. This can be caused by an overactive detrusor or by hypersensitivity.
- Overflow incontinence: this occurs as a result of retention of urine, which is often caused by prostate enlargement or urethral strictures.
- Reflex incontinence: individuals with a disruption to the simple reflex arc may suffer with this kind of incontinence due to the loss of sensation.
- Enuresis: this term refers to the involuntary loss of urine. It is commonly associated with incontinence when the person is asleep, and is called nocturnal enuresis.
- Immobility incontinence: people who would normally be continent but due to circumstances such as a pre-existing disease or disability preventing them from going to an appropriate place to pass urine, may experience this type of incontinence.

Once it has been determined exactly which type of incontinence is being experienced, the appropriate treatment plan can be decided on.

Sociological influences in continence

Incontinence is to some degree a hidden problem among the general public, with a reluctance by many to admit their incontinence and subsequently search for treatment. In many cases, there is a trigger for individuals to seek help and advice, and this usually arises from social and personal interaction. Such triggers include:

- interpersonal crises
- perception of interference of the problem with social or personal relationships
- pressure from others to consult a doctor
- perception of interference of the problem with vocational or physical activity
- reaching of a personal deadline for symptoms to be resolved.

Many people feel that incontinence is a major source of embarrassment or shame, rather than a signal for them to seek medical help. In this situation, the bladder dysfunction is seen in terms of its social constraints only.

Treatment of incontinence

Once the type of incontinence has been established, there are a number of treatments available. These include pelvic floor exercises, bladder training, anticholinergic drugs, CISC, dietary advice, the resolving of underlying medical conditions and surgical intervention.

Pelvic floor exercises

These are intended to increase the strength of the levator ani muscles and to evoke their contraction without increasing abdominal pressure (Figures 5.1 and 5.2).

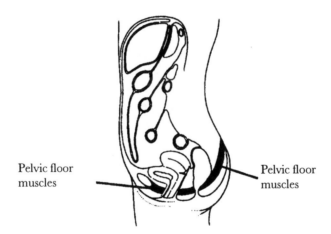

Pelvic floor muscles — Pelvic floor muscles

Figure 5.1 Female pelvic floor muscles.

Bladder retraining

If an individual has urge incontinence, bladder retraining combined with anticholinergic drugs (such as oxybutynin) would be the treatment of choice. The bladder is taught to increase its capacity and therefore lengthen the intervals between voiding.

The patient is advised to refrain from voiding for a few more minutes between the signal to void and going to void. When the lengthened time between each void is achieved, new goals are set.

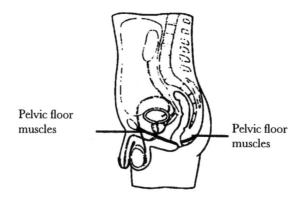

Pelvic floor
muscles

Pelvic floor
muscles

Figure 5.2 Male pelvic floor muscles.

Clean intermittent self-catheterization

Patients with an atonic bladder or dysnergia would find this treatment
beneficial. (See Chapter 11 for details concerning this procedure.)

Surgical intervention

In some cases of stress incontinence, women will need to undergo
surgical intervention. These operations are carried out either per
vagina or via a suprapubic route. The suprapubic route is the
preferred choice, where the bladder neck is hitched up or supported
with sutures. The most common operation is known as a colposuspension, where the paravaginal fascia is sutured to the ileopectinal
ligament. There are two approaches – either a Stamey colposuspension or a Birch colposuspension.

Nursing care post-colposuspension

Postoperatively, the nurse needs to record vital signs on a regular
basis.

The patient will have a vaginal pack in situ, which will be
removed 48 hours after surgery.

Urinary output needs to be recorded and observed. Women who
have undergone this type of operation are at real risk of developing
urinary retention and may need to be catheterized.

The urologist will be interested in knowing how the patient feels
about their continence postoperatively – are they dry, or occasionally
wet?

Abdominal sutures will need to be removed at the usual time of 7–10 days, with the nurse taking care of the wound and re-dressing it as appropriate.

In cases where this operation fails, the patient may need to be taught CISC, or opt for further reconstructive bladder surgery.

Other treatments for incontinence

In some cases, the individual will require more traditional treatments, such as pad and pants, urinary sheath or long-term catheterization. The nurse needs to remember that each person and each case is unique. Referral to a continence advisor is appropriate in order to attain up-to-date knowledge of continence, the products available and treatment choices.

Other surgical treatment choices

Enterocystoplasty

Patients with a small-capacity bladder may benefit from enlarging the capacity using a piece of resected bowel to enhance the bladder size.

Prior to surgery, the patient should be taught CISC in case they need to perform this postoperatively.

Preparation will include a fluids-only diet for 48 hours preoperatively, and use of aperients to clear and cleanse the large bowel.

During surgery, a section of bowel is removed and opened out so that it can be sutured into the form of a sheet of tissue. This is then sutured on to the opened bladder to create a larger reservoir.

Postoperative care

The patient will have an IV infusion and a PCA or epidural. There will be a urethral and suprapubic catheter, which should be monitored for their output (it does not matter which catheter drains, as long as there is drainage. Usually there will be a switch between the two catheters when one drains and the other doesn't).

Oral fluids will be introduced when bowel sounds are heard.

Some patients experience the problem of mucus (secreted by the anastomosed bowel), which can block the catheters and cause either retention or bypassing. This is treated by performing gentle twice-daily saline bladder washouts through the catheters. It has also been reported that if the patient drinks cranberry juice, this can reduce the amount of secretions (Lever 1996).

Prior to discharge home, the patient will be taught to perform bladder washouts. They will be allowed home and subsequently brought back into hospital 6 weeks later for a cystogram and removal of catheters. The cystogram will ensure that there is no leakage from the suture line.

Endoscopic bladder transection

In some cases, the patient may benefit from an enlarged bladder capacity. This can be achieved by performing an endoscopic bladder transection, where a cystoscope is used in order to create a deep cut into the bladder mucosa thus increasing the possible bladder volume.

Nursing care postoperatively

This includes the care of an individual with a catheter in situ. After a short period of time (e.g. 24 hours) the catheter should be removed and the output volumes of the patient recorded.

Artificial sphincters

Individuals with defective sphincters (diagnosed in urodynamics) may well benefit from the insertion of an artificial sphincter. This requires the patient to undergo a general anaesthetic for the insertion of the sphincter and mechanism.

The cuff of the sphincter is fixed around the bladder neck and a reservoir mechanism is inserted in the abdominal wall. The sphincter is kept in the inactive state at this stage.

Postoperative care

This includes the care of individuals with drains and catheters. A PCA or epidural will be in place for pain control.

Tuition is needed for catheter care in the community, along with community nursing support on discharge.

After 6 weeks has elapsed postoperatively, the patient should be brought back into hospital for catheter removal. The consultant will then activate the sphincter and instruct the patient in its use.

Following this, care regarding output volume measurements is needed, because the patient has a great risk of going into retention.

Bladder stones

People presenting with bladder stones tend to experience pain on walking rather than sitting down (Blandy 1991). They can usually be seen on plain KUB X-ray.

Treatment

In many cases, the stone can be treated with litholapaxy (where the stone is surgically crushed), and sometimes by using the lithotripter. Extreme cases, however, will need a suprapubic lithotomy where the bladder is opened and the stone retrieved.

Cystitis

Cystitis is an inflammation of the bladder, characterized by frequency, urgency and dysuria. It is usually caused by organisms entering the bladder through the urethra, but can also be associated with certain drug therapies and post-radiation therapy (Watson 1979).

Usually, the inflammation is confined to the mucosa and submucosa, which are also oedematous. Haematuria may be present, as well as organisms.

Prior to commencing treatment, the patient should provide a mid-stream sample (or catheter sample) of urine for culture and sensitivity. The infection can then be treated with the most appropriate therapy.

Chapter 6
The prostate

PHILIP DOWNEY

Benign prostatic hyperplasia

Approximately 2.5 million men in the UK have lower urinary tract symptoms due to benign prostatic hyperplasia (BPH) (Garraway et al. 1991). The attitudes towards this condition appear to be changing, due to increased awareness and particularly of the bothersome symptoms that can have an impact on the quality of life. However, many men are still likely to suffer in silence with prostate problems.

The gland slowly increases in size from birth to puberty, when it undertakes a rapid growth spurt. The size it attains by the age of 30 remains stable until the male reaches his forties, when enlargement can occur.

The normal, healthy prostate has no true lobes. As the gland deforms by benign nodular hypertrophy the lateral and middle lobes become evident (Blandy 1991) (Figure 6.1). Over the age of 40, most men have some degree of BPH and studies suggest that one in three will develop BPH over the age of 50 (Garraway et al. 1991), so making BPH so common an occurrence that the absence of it in the older man is regarded as abnormal. The financial cost of BPH to the NHS has been calculated as between £62 million and £91 million (estimated as 92.38 million to 135.59 million ECUs; exchange rate = 1.49 ECUs to £1, June 1998) per annum (Drummond et al. 1993).

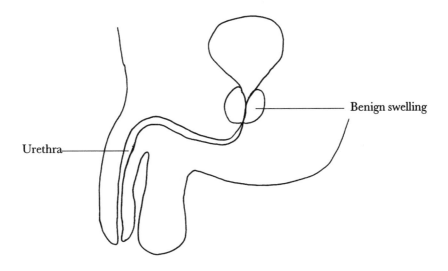

Figure 6.1 Benign prostatic hyperplasia.

Once enlargement occurs, many men will experience some degree of nocturia, frequency and urgency. It is at this stage that a 'watchful waiting' approach may be adopted, using a symptom score as a guide to how bothersome the prostate has become (Cockett et al. 1993) (Figure 6.2). However, the size of prostate enlargement is unrelated to the degree of urethral obstruction. The smallest prostate may cause the worst outflow obstruction.

With increased outflow obstruction, the detrusor responds by becoming stronger. Initially, the wall of the bladder will become thickened. At first, the increased power of the detrusor keeps the bladder empty, and the flow rate appears to be maintained. There may be some frequency and urgency at this stage, but the stream may appear to be unaffected. After a while, the detrusor will weaken and the bladder no longer empties itself. As a result, the residual volume of urine grows and becomes a potential focus for infection.

As time passes, the residual volume will become so large that the individual can suffer with chronic retention. The bladder wall by this stage tends to be fibrous tissue. The ureter will become dilated with hydronephrosis due to back pressure, and renal failure becomes a reality.

International Prostate Symptom Score PSS

	Not at all	Less than 1 time in 5	Less than half the time	About half the time	More than half the time	Almost always	Your score
Patient Name:							
Date:							
1. Incomplete emptying Over the past month, how often have you had a sensation of not emptying your bladder completely after you finish urinating?	0	1	2	3	4	5	
2. Frequency Over the past month, how often have you had to urinate again less than two hours after you finished urinating?	0	1	2	3	4	5	
3. Intermittency Over the past month, how often have you found you stopped and started again several times when you urinated?	0	1	2	3	4	5	
4. Urgency Over the past month, how often have you found it difficult to postpone urination?	0	1	2	3	4	5	

	None	1 time	2 times	3 times	4 times	5 times or more
5. Weak stream Over the past month, how often have you had a weak urinary stream?	0	1	2	3	4	5
6. Straining Over the past month, how often have you had to push or strain to begin urination?	0	1	2	3	4	5
7. Nocturia Over the past month, how many times did you most typically get up to urinate from the time you went to bed at night until the time you got up in the morning?	0	1	2	3	4	5
Total I-PSS Score						

Figure 6.2 International prostate symptom score.

Medical/surgical intervention

A man with bladder outflow obstruction will need some form of medical intervention before the detrusor is grossly affected. The main symptoms that make a patient visit the GP are usually frequency and poor flow rate. Outflow incontinence due to chronic retention may be another cause.

Most medical staff or nurse specialists will perform a digital rectal examination (DRE). However, this can appear to be misleading in some cases. A flow rate test followed by bladder scan to detect the residual volume of urine would be most informative.

Transurethral resection of prostate (TURP)

The most common way of treating BPH is to perform a transurethral resection of prostate. It is performed using a cysto-scope, which is passed up the penis, usually under general anaesthetic. It is passed up to the prostate via the urethra, and leaves no visible scars and causes very little pain.

Nursing care post-TURP

More than likely, the patient will have an IV infusion. A catheter will be in situ, with a 0.9% saline irrigation system in place also. There is usually haematuria. This solution and the catheter should only remain in place for a couple of days, with the catheter being removed at midnight on the day of choice (Downey et al. 1997).

Transurethral incision of prostate (TUIP)

This procedure has been performed for over 20 years, but is only recently starting to be favoured by UK surgeons. It involves making incisions into the prostatic tissue to create an enlarged lumen to the prostatic urethra. This helps to relieve bladder outflow obstruction without actually resecting the prostatic tissue.

Individual patients with a small but bothersome prostate would be ideal candidates for this procedure. It would also be indicated if the patient is young or middle-aged.

TUIP can be performed under either general anaesthetic or local anaesthetic (the local anaesthetic being an option in a day-case setting). This treatment option has proved to be as successful as TURP in relieving symptoms and actually appears to provide a longer time span between repeating the procedure (Lepor et al. 1992).

Nursing care post-TUIP

Nursing care is concerned with catheter care postoperatively. The catheter (if present) should be removed at midnight 48 hours after the procedure (Downey et al. 1997).

In some cases, a catheter may not be present, in which case, the nursing care will focus around fluid intake/output monitoring.

In all situations, the patient's vital signs need to be recorded at regular intervals in order to observe for any signs of haemorrhage from the internal wound site.

Laser therapy

This method of treatment is increasing in popularity. The patient undergoes laser therapy in a similar method to a flexicystoscopy. The laser is aimed at the prostate, and treatment is commenced. It would appear that this form of treatment is able to be used in day-case surgery, because the patient does not suffer with any bleeding point. But usually an overnight stay is needed.

The patient will have a catheter in situ immediately postoperatively. This will be removed the morning after surgery, or preferably at midnight the same day (Downey et al. 1997). As the prostate sloughs away, the patient is not usually at risk of retention, and will experience only a 'clouding' of the urine as the most noticeable symptom. Within 2–3 weeks the prostate will return to its normal pre-hypertrophied state, with minimal additional symptoms.

Nursing care post-laser therapy

Nursing management is minimal in this near day-case situation. Vital signs may be recorded postoperatively, and additional advice and support given to the patient.

Transurethral needle abliteration (TUNA)

TUNA is another alternative being discussed widely among urological surgeons. It is performed by insertion of a needle into the prostate gland, and the circulation of very-high-frequency radio waves. This treatment is meant to be used in day-case surgery. As yet its success rate is unclear, however, it would appear to be relatively successful.

A catheter may be needed in the early stages of postoperative recovery if the patient had previously needed one, until the prostate shrinks in size.

Nursing care post-TUNA

Nursing involvement is again minimal in this day-case surgery. Advice and assistance may be needed by the patient, along with education regarding catheter maintenance.

Transwave thermotherapy (T3)

This is currently still in the research stage. A probe similar to a catheter is inserted into the urethra until the thermal area of the probe sits within the prostate capsule. In addition, a rectal probe is used to monitor the temperature from the urethral probe.

Microwave energy is then passed via the urethral probe as indicated by protocol. The aim of this treatment is to shrink the prostate using heat.

Nursing care post-T3

While this has only been researched in Liverpool and Colchester in the UK, it would appear that nursing involvement remains minimal, except for during the procedure itself. Careful monitoring of the equipment in use is extremely important during treatment.

Prostatic stent insertion

A prostatic stent is a small coil-like catheter which sits in the prostatic urethra. There is no visible catheter, and the patient should be issued with a card in case of emergencies. Due to the nature of this catheter, there should not be any attempt to insert a urethral catheter in a patient with a prostatic stent. If the patient is experiencing retention of urine, a suprapubic catheter would be indicated.

Only in rare cases is it possible for an experienced urologist to insert a urethral catheter.

Nursing care post-prostatic stent

Initially the patient may experience incontinence following prostatic stent insertion. This is usually due to the stent becoming embedded into the prostatic urethra over a period of time. Nursing management involves care of the potentially incontinent patient, or the patient experiencing retention of urine.

Chemical intervention

When surgery is not the preferred treatment of choice, there are a number of options available in the form of medication.

Alpha blockers

Doxazosin may be prescribed. This is a selective beta blocker. In individuals with BPH, doxazosin works by relaxing smooth muscle. As a result, it helps by increasing the flow rate and thereby relieving the symptoms associated with obstruction. It can take up to 2 weeks to achieve maximum response with this drug (Editorial 1995).

Anti-androgens

Finasteride works by inhibiting the metabolism of testosterone and dihydrotestosterone. The effect of this is to reduce prostate size over an average 6-month period and therefore relieve the symptoms of obstruction. A better flow rate is produced as a result (Editorial 1995).

The risk of incontinence following treatment for BPH

In rare cases, the individual may experience continence problems (Carney et al. 1995). It would appear that with the new-style treatments, such as TUNA and laser therapy, the prospects of incontinence are negligible.

Initially, continence problems should be treated by encouraging pelvic floor exercises and the immediate use of continence aids. Problems that are unrelieved by pelvic floor exercises should be referred to a continence advisory nurse, who can give expert help.

Effects of treatment on sexuality

Retrograde ejaculation occurs in nearly all men who have undergone TURP (Murphy and Malloy 1987). In most cases this is not a problem due to the age of the patient (usually over 60), because they feel that their days of fathering children are over. However, it is an important reason for informed consent (UKCC 1996), as some people may feel that their fertility is still important despite their age. Most men report that they feel no difference in their sex lives and are happy with the feeling that they experience, because their climax feels normal (Carney et al. 1995).

A small number of men will complain of impotence following a TURP. If this occurs, the individual may need referral to an andrology clinic for examination and advice. In some cases, it is possible for individuals to become impotent through worry and anxiety. Andrology services may help provide the answers to these men.

Cancer of the prostate

Cancer of the prostate is the third most common malignancy in Western men (Brewster et al. 1994). Within England, the Department of Health (DoH) episode statistics 1994–5 show that 24 922 men have been diagnosed as having a malignant neoplasm, with 21 645 being over the age of 65 (DoH 1995). Autopsy reports have also shown that latent prostate cancer was found in 95% of men who were older than 90 years of age at the times of their deaths, suggesting that cancerous changes may be part of the ageing process (Piemme 1988).

Adenocarcinomas account for more than 90% of tumours, although other types do occur, including small cell, transitional cell, melanoma and sarcoma. They are usually found in the peripheral and transitional zones of the prostate, with the peripheral zone accounting for more than 70% of prostatic gland tissue.

Clinical presentation

Most patients will normally present with signs and symptoms resembling outflow obstruction – very similar to the signs and symptoms of BPH. However, there is often a relatively shorter history of symptoms, namely for months rather than years, and occasional haematuria.

In individuals with outflow obstruction, the priority remains to relieve the obstruction. Those with acute or chronic retention will require catheterization and possibly a channel TURP to help alleviate the symptoms.

Occasionally, patients may present with symptoms related to metastatic spread or lymphatic involvement, such as either pain or oedema. Approximately 10–15% of men will present with symptoms relating only to their metastases (usually bony secondaries).

Assessment of the tumour is made using a number of methods, namely: DRE, prostate-specific antigen (PSA), transrectal ultrasound and transrectal biopsy.

Grading and staging

Grading of the tumour is based on the degree of differentiation or anaplasia of the tumour cells. The Gleason score (Gleason and Mellinger 1974) appears to be a good predictor of prognosis, because of a strong correlation between the histological score and the presence of identifiable metastases (Sagalowsky et al. 1982).

Medical/surgical management

Transurethral resection of prostate (TURP)

This is normally performed when the tumour is small and confined to the capsule. It is performed in the same manner as TURP for BPH.

Radical prostatectomy

This procedure requires the surgeon to dissect adjacent structures while excising the pelvic lymph nodes, seminal vesicles and the prostate gland. Protection of the bundles during the procedure contributes to the preservation of sexual function and urinary continence, commonly a complication of radical prostatectomy (Walsh 1992).

Nursing care post-radical prostatectomy

Nursing care will include interventions that promote comfort, facilitate urinary output, support wound healing, maintain fluid balance and prevent postoperative complications.

The patient will have an IV infusion, PCA (or epidural), a three-way irrigating catheter and one or two wound drains. The PCA or epidural will be removed after 3–4 days, once a reduction is seen in the amount of analgesia being required. The patient will then be converted to either intramuscular or oral analgesia. The IV infusion will be discontinued once bowel sounds are heard, and providing electrolyte balance is maintained and diet can be tolerated.

Wound drains need to be observed, and pelvic drains will ooze a serous fluid until about day 4 or 5 postoperatively.

It is usual for patients who have had a radical prostatectomy to be discharged home after 10–14 days with a hydrogel catheter in situ. The patient will then need to be readmitted 3–4 weeks later for an overnight stay in order to perform a trial without catheter. Ideally the catheter should be removed at midnight on the day of readmission (Downey et al. 1997).

Hormone manipulation

One of the most active procedures at reducing the intensity of the disease is manipulation of the hormones that supply the tumour, because nearly 85% of prostate cancers are androgen-dependent (Lind and Nakao 1990). As treatment is designed to reduce the amount of circulating hormones (Taylor 1991), the goal is to block hormone production to arrest the prostate cancer.

Men undertaking manipulation must be advised that there will be some body image changes, and that it will also make them impotent. As a result, informed consent is essential (UKCC 1996).

Bilateral subcapsular orchidectomy

This is the surgical removal of the inside of the testes, which are responsible for the production of testosterone. It is irreversible and can have a considerable psychological impact on the patient. The testicular shell remains intact.

Nursing care post-subcapsular orchidectomy

Nursing care includes care of a scrotal wound, ensuring that the wound is hygienically clean. It is also important for these men to wear a well-padded scrotal support until the wounds are properly healed. Sutures will dissolve approximately 7–10 days postoperatively.

Oestrogen therapy

Oestrogen inhibits circulating testosterone, reducing the amount of gonadotrophins secreted by the pituitary. Effects of this treatment are reversible if stopped within 2 years.

Nursing care

This includes ensuring medication compliance.

Anti-androgens

Anti-androgens act on specific sites in the prostate cells to inhibit the binding of dihydrotestosterone and testosterone to receptor proteins. They also block androgens produced by the adrenal glands.

Nursing care

This includes ensuring compliance with medication.

Gonadotrophin-releasing hormone analogues

These cause stimulation and suppression of pituitary gonadotrophin, which then results in a reduction of testosterone levels. It can be administered by monthly or 3-monthly depot pellet. Once commenced, this treatment is given for the rest of the patient's life, or until another treatment is adopted.

Nursing care

This is mainly concerned with care of the injection site.

Radiotherapy and chemotherapy

Radiotherapy and chemotherapy have only a small part to play in the treatment of prostate cancer. Chemotherapy may offer palliative treatment for men with hormone-resistant disease, and it appears to have little part to play in the treatment of hormone-escaped prostate cancer (Klimaszewski and Karlowicz 1995).

Prostatitis

The term prostatitis means that the prostate gland is inflamed, and it usually presents in either acute or (the more common experience) chronic variations. Acute prostatitis is virtually always caused by bacterial infection and chronic prostatitis is most commonly non-bacterial, but can also sometimes be caused by infection (Kirby 1997).

Acute bacterial prostatitis

Acute prostatitis may well be precipitated by urethral instrumentation or meatal inoculation during sexual intercourse (Kirby 1997), trauma, bladder outflow obstruction or from prostatic massage in individuals with chronic prostatitis (Giroux 1995).

Patients with acute bacterial prostatitis usually complain of sudden chills, fever, lower back pain, perineal pain and acute onset of urinary tract symptoms. General malaise also tends to develop. If DRE is performed, it reveals a swollen, tender prostate and the examination will be extremely uncomfortable for the patient. Midstream urine tends to culture *Escherichia coli* in approximately 80% of individuals (Kirby 1997).

Treatment of acute bacterial prostatitis

Patients with this condition usually respond well to antibiotic therapy. Urethral instrumentation (i.e. urethral catheterization) is not recommended, and if the patient should experience urinary retention, then suprapubic catheterization would be indicated (Giroux 1995).

Nursing care

The nurse's role involves the administration of medication and monitoring of urinary output – observing for its depletion or signs of acute retention.

Vital signs need to be recorded regularly to monitor the course of the condition.

Psychological support may be needed by individuals who have experienced transient impotence as a result of the acute prostatitis. The patient may need reassurance that this problem will correct itself once treatment is completed.

Prostatic abscess

It is possible for acute prostatitis to progress to the formation of prostatic abscesses, although this is unusual. The main causative organism is *E. coli*, and occasionally it is caused by *Staphylococcus aureus* or *Pseudomonas*.

The men most at risk of this condition appear to be those with diabetes, chronic renal failure or immunosuppressed individuals.

Diagnosis is usually made using computerized tomography (CT) scanning, because transrectal ultrasound would be too painful to perform.

Treatment of prostatic abscess

Prostatic abscess is usually treated with high doses of antibiotics. It may be necessary to aspirate the abscess under ultrasound control. The most effective way of treating this condition would appear to be the transurethral incision of the abscess using a resectoscope under general anaesthetic.

Nursing care

This is mainly concerned with the administration of antibiotic therapy in the early stages. It is important that vital signs are recorded on a regular basis to monitor the effectiveness of medication being administered.

If the individual needs to go to theatre, the nurse will be concerned with normal postoperative care.

Chronic bacterial prostatitis

Chronic bacterial prostatitis can develop after an episode of inadequate treatment of acute prostatitis, or following urethral obstruction, or indeed without any previous history (Giroux 1995). Other contributory factors to this condition include: urethral inoculation by pathogenic vaginal bacteria, unprotected penetrative rectal intercourse, indwelling urethral catheter or condom drainage device, and possibly an untreated urinary tract infection following TURP (Kirby 1997). Only 5% of men with chronic prostatitis have acquired the condition through bacterial infection of the prostate.

The main feature of chronic bacterial prostatitis is relapsing urinary tract infection, and some men complain of perineal pain and possibly outflow symptoms. DRE will yield little information, with the prostate feeling somewhat normal, indurated or even boggy. Accurate diagnosis is made following a lower tract localization test, performed by:

1   initial void of urine
2   mid-stream specimen of urine
3   prostatic massage and production of prostatic secretions
4   first void following massage.

All samples are cultured.

Treatment of chronic bacterial prostatitis

This treatment is long-term and can be a source of frustration for the patient. Antibiotics such as ciprofloxacin are advisable for this condition. It is not clear how long the duration of treatment should be, but an average of 6 weeks is usually recommended (Kirby 1997).

Nursing care

Nursing care involves the administration of medication and the education of the patient regarding the need to continue therapy once discharged from hospital.

Care will also include psychological support of the patient, who may well feel frustrated with his treatment and response rate to the medication – due to the length of the course of treatment.

Chronic non-bacterial prostatitis

This is the most common form of prostatitis, and yet its etiology remains unknown at present. This means that its treatment can sometimes be difficult. Chronic non-bacterial prostatitis appears to be either an infectious disease caused by organisms such as *Chlamydia trachomatis* and *Mycoplasma hominis* (i.e. possibly through sexually transmitted diseases), or a non-infectious form of inflammation.

Diagnosis of this condition rests on the symptoms of perineal pain and varying urinary and sexual dysfunction. There would be no history of bladder infection (Kirby 1997). A colour doppler image is useful to assist with diagnosis on transrectal ultrasound because this would indicate inflammatory changes.

Treatment of chronic non-bacterial prostatitis

Treatment for chronic non-bacterial prostatitis is difficult. Some individuals respond well to antibiotic therapy, and therefore a trial with antibiotics is recommended. If specific organisms such as *Chlamydia trachomatis* are present, then these should be treated accordingly.

The patient may achieve comfort if prescribed anti-inflammatory drug therapy such as ibuprofen.

Some patients find that therapeutic prostatic massage helps to relieve the symptoms. In conjunction with this, the patient may find that increased sexual activity or masturbation affords some relief of the congested prostate. It should be remembered that if this course of action is adopted, the patient needs to be aware of the need to use a condom if he has *Chlamydia* present, in order to protect his partner from infection (Giroux 1995).

Nursing care

The nurse remains responsible for the administration of medication – antibiotics and analgesics. Vital signs will continue to be monitored on a regular basis.

Prostatodynia

Prostatodynia means 'painful prostate', and is the presence of symptoms of prostatitis in the absence of physical findings. It is extremely difficult to distinguish this from either chronic or non-bacterial prostatitis. The condition is seen in young men between 25 and 45 years. Etiology is uncertain, but various suggestions have been made. One suggestion is that the symptoms arise from tension within the pelvic floor, and others include incomplete relaxation of the bladder neck with abnormal narrowing of the urethra at the external urethral sphincter (Giroux 1995).

Diagnosis is difficult, due to symptoms common to non-bacterial prostatitis. There is no history of urinary tract infection and no abnormality on DRE.

Treatment of prostatodynia

It has been reported that in some cases patients will respond to alpha blockers such as doxazosin or alfuzocin. If these drugs are successful, there is no definite duration of treatment.

As with non-bacterial prostatitis, symptomatic relief may be achieved with prostatic massage.

Nursing care

Nursing care includes medication compliance and psychological support. Provision of warm baths for the patient to sit in may also assist in patient recovery.

Chapter 7
The penis and urethra

PHILIP DOWNEY

Penile carcinoma

The incidence of penile carcinoma is rare. It tends to occur in men between the ages of 20 and 60 years, with a mean age at diagnosis of 58 years (Crawford and Dawkins 1988; Burgers et al. 1992). As with other cancers, there are documented risk factors, including late or lack of circumcision and poor hygiene (Nichols 1988). The suggestion that poor hygiene is linked with this cancer is made, because smegma has been associated with carcinogenesis in animals, although the specific carcinogenic compounds of smegma have not been identified (Flannery 1992).

Within England and Wales, the mortality statistics show 93 deaths from malignant cancer of the penis. Within a 10-year period from 1981 to 1990, 240 new cases were diagnosed in Norway, and less than 1% of male cancers were penile carcinoma in the USA (Crawford and Dawkins 1988).

Penile cancer can often appear as small pimples or warts or a nodule on the shaft of the penis. As it progresses, primary carcinoma of the penis will spread via the lymphatics and more than half of the patients with this condition will present with some form of lymphadenopathy. This could be either cancer of the lymph nodes or inflammation due to infection of the lesion (Nichols 1988) (Table 7.1).

Metastatic spread is present in one third of all patients with penile cancer when the diagnosis is actually made (Grabstald 1990).

Table 7.1 Staging of penile carcinoma

Stage	Presentation
I	Cancer is confined to foreskin or glans
II	Cancer has begun to invade shaft of the penis
III	Cancer has begun to invade the scrotum
IV	Inguinal nodes are involved

Distant metastases from this condition are uncommon because they appear late in the disease process, and can involve bone, lung or liver (Nichols 1988).

The most common type of cancer of the penis is squamous cell carcinoma, with 95% of malignancies being this type. It can originate anywhere on the penis, with 48% being on the glans and 21% on the prepuce (Burgers et al. 1992).

Medical management

All men presenting with this condition need to have a medical–surgical assessment performed to evaluate the lesion. This includes a biopsy to ascertain the extent of the malignancy and its histology.

The treatment of penile cancer is selected on the extent of its invasion. Surgery, chemotherapy and/or radiotherapy all have pros and cons. If the cancer is located at the foreskin, and is mainly a non-invasive carcinoma, circumcision is the treatment of choice. However, this is associated with a recurrence rate of 50% (Schell-hammer et al. 1992).

If the cancer is located on the glans or distal third of the shaft, and it is between 2 cm and 5 cm in diameter, then partial penile amputation is indicated (Crawford and Dawkins 1988; Johnson and Lo 1987). A total penectomy would be indicated if the cancer originated on the proximal shaft of the penis. This treatment renders the patient unable to stand while urinating.

Nursing care

Post-circumcision
The nurse should record vital signs at regular intervals, observing for signs of haemorrhage. Observation of the wound should be recorded at the same time.

The day after theatre, the dressing will be removed and replaced with a non-stick dressing such as paraffin jelly gauze and dry dressing. The nurse must educate the patient about keeping the wound clean and advise him that the sutures will dissolve in about 7–10 days.

The nurse will also need to inform the patient that he should refrain from any sexual activity until the wound is fully healed, i.e. up to 14 days postoperatively.

Post-penile amputation (or partial amputation)
On return to the ward, the patient will have a urinary catheter and wound drain. Pain will most probably be controlled using a PCA. He will be kept hydrated using an IV infusion, until it becomes apparent that he can tolerate oral fluids and that there is no need for a blood transfusion (following surgery in such a vascularized area).

Drains and catheter will be removed over a period of 2 weeks. The nurse must observe for signs of urinary retention. Ideally, the catheter should be removed at midnight on the day of choice for this very reason (Downey et al. 1997).

Sutures will be removed approximately 10 days postoperatively.

Psychological impact of cancer of the penis

Once penile cancer has been diagnosed, feelings such as anxiety, shock and a sense of loss will be experienced by the patient. It will have a significant impact on his self-image and his male status in society.

The patient who has a partner and an active sex life may not adjust very well. Both the patient and his partner need to be given time to come to terms with this condition and how it will impact on their lives. Many men feel that penile amputation is surgical removal of their masculinity – in much the same way that women feel mastectomy removes their femininity. The man and his partner need to be given the opportunity to express their fears and anxieties. This may even manifest in the man becoming an extremely aggressive and even verbally abusive patient – a factor that all nurses need to be aware of. These mood swings and altered behaviour patterns will tend to disappear once the man and his partner start to come to terms with the condition and its treatment.

Just as the patient need psychological support, the partners of these people will also need help in understanding other ways of expressing love for their partner, and that there can be a loving relationship without the need for penetrative sex. Nurses are in a position to advise and help these people and their partners in an attempt to minimize the psychological trauma.

Phimosis

Phimosis is the condition where a man is unable to retract his foreskin over the glans. It can be caused by infection or trauma, and usually tends to be highlighted when it interferes with sexual intercourse. In these cases, men complain of pain or bleeding during sex.

Medical intervention

The surgeon may decide to perform either a dorsal slit in the foreskin, or a complete circumcision. The dorsal slit will allow the man to retract his foreskin as normal.

Nursing care post-circumcision / dorsal slit

See pp 99–100.

Paraphimosis

Paraphimosis occurs when the foreskin is contricted behind the glans, so that it cannot be replaced to its normal position. It causes compression of the dorsal veins and lymphatics of the distal end of the penis, increasing the oedema. It can happen after the man has washed under the foreskin as part of his hygiene routine, or after intercourse, if the retracted foreskin is not replaced.

This condition is also common with poor urinary catheter insertion technique, if the nurse or doctor performing the technique fails to return the foreskin to its normal position.

Medical/nursing management

Paraphimosis is classed as a medical emergency. If the foreskin is not replaced as soon as possible, the more difficult it is to rectify the situation. Delayed action means that the arterial supply to the glans will be blocked and gangrene of the glans is a real possibility.

The reduction of oedematous fluid is the first step in treating this condition – and can be performed by the nurse without medical instruction. It is performed by the application of pressure on the glans for several minutes before attempting to reposition the fore-skin. The use of ice packs may also be of benefit.

Reduction of paraphimosis is a painful procedure, and if it remains unsuccessful medical staff need to be informed. A decision will then be made regarding the need to perform a circumcision.

Peyronies disease

The cause of this condition remains unknown. In Peyronies disease, a hard plaque of fibrous tissue forms in the Buck's fascia or in the septum between the corpora. Similar lumps can be found in the ear lobes, the palmar fascia (i.e. Dupuytren's contracture) and in the retroperitoneal tissue (i.e. idiopathic retroperitoneal fibrosis) (Blandy 1991).

The resultant effect of the laying down of the plaques means that the filling of the corpus cavernosum is affected, and will create a curvature of the penis upon erection (Figure 7.1). Severe curvature (up to and including a 90 degree bend) will make it impossible for the man to engage in penetrative sex.

Surgical maintenance

The usual 'cure' for Peyronies disease is to operate on the patient (normally under general anaesthetic). During this procedure the

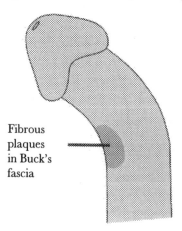

Fibrous
plaques
in Buck's
fascia

Figure 7.1 Peyronies disease.

surgeon will create an artificial erection by injecting 0.9% saline into the corpus cavernosum. The urologist is then able to see the extent and angle of curvature. At this point, it is then possible to perform a Nesbit's plication.

The Nesbit's plication is performed by the removal of several tucks of Buck's fascia on the opposite side to the curve. It is done until the penis appears straight. The patient needs to be aware that this operation will reduce the length of the erect penis, due to the necessary removal of healthy tissue on the unaffected side of the curve. They should also be made aware that this will not necessarily affect their sex lives.

Nursing care

Nursing care is mainly concerned with the general care of the post-operative patient. The nurse needs to monitor the wound site initially for signs of bleeding.

The patient should be advised to refrain from sexual activity until the internal and external sutures are fully healed, i.e. up to 14 days postoperatively. Both sets of sutures are normally soluble.

The patient needs to be made aware of the need for good hygiene and general wound care principles.

Penile fracture

Penile fracture actually refers to the rupture of the tunica albuginea when the penis is erect. A loud snapping sound can be heard and felt at the time of the injury. This is then followed by a rapid onset of pain and oedema (Reilly 1995).

Fracture of the penis can occur during rigorous sexual intercourse, when the penis may be abnormally bent. It may also occur during sleep, or even from a blow to the erect penis.

In some cases, nurse specialists are now finding that a number of patients who present at the impotence clinic and who are treated using a vacuum device may also experience penile fracture. This is due to the non-ridigity of the penis below the constricting elastic band. Therefore, with an inherent lack of support throughout the whole of the corpus cavernosum, there is a possibility for the penis to bend abnormally.

Medical treatment

Penile fracture can be treated conservatively or through surgical management. Managing the condition in a conservative manner will include catheterization, cool packs and compression bandaging.

Surgical treatment requires the haematoma to be removed and a repair to the tunica albuginea to be carried out.

Scandinavian studies show that normal erectile function usually returns within 2 days of intervention, and that the man is able to return to coitus at around 13 days after treatment. Some men have also reported a slight curvature of the erect penis (like in Peyronies disease, but not as severe); this does not generally stop the man returning to his usual sexual activity (Uygur et al. 1997).

Nursing care

This usually centres around care of the postoperative patient – if the patient is operated on. The nurse should maintain regular monitoring of vital signs in case of bleeding, and observation of fluid intake/output.

Psychological support of the patient is also important. The man and his partner need to be able to express their worries regarding sexual relationships and practices. Each individual needs to be reassured that this is a temporary situation, and that their lives will return to normal within a few days or weeks.

Penile strangulation

This occurs when something is placed around the penis and creates a strangulation effect. It is possibly caused by incorrectly applied condom continence devices, string or bands used for the purpose of enhancing erection for sexual pleasure.

The longer the condition is left, the greater the possibility of severe necrosis and gangrene. It is quite possible for the patient who delays treatment (for maybe 24 hours or more) to experience long-term effects from this condition, including severe nerve damage rendering the man incapable of achieving erection again.

Medical involvement will include the removal of the cause of strangulation. Debridement of the necrotic tissue may be required, but is not routinely performed.

Nursing care

Nurses need to observe the patient's urinary output – with a swollen, oedematous penis it is quite possible for the patient to go into acute urinary retention.

The nurse also needs to record if the patient feels altered sensation and or pain. Analgesics should be given as prescribed.

If the cause of the condition was the man's sexual behaviour, then the nurse has a role in educating him (and his partner) of the dangers of using rings around the penis. They should be reassured that once the tissue returns to normal, in most cases, full function will return to the penis.

Urethral trauma in men

This may be caused by a number of accidents, and is usually from a blunt trauma. It can also be caused by surgical intervention (i.e. performing a cystoscopy) or by self-manipulation.

Urethral trauma is classified into two distinct categories, namely anterior urethral injury (involving the penile urethra, caused by straddle-type injury, instrumentation such as inflating a catheter balloon in the wrong place, or the insertion of objects into the urethra for sexual pleasure) and posterior urethral injury (which tends to occur in conjunction with pelvic fracture) (Table 7.2).

Table 7.2 Causes of urethral trauma

Anterior injuries	Posterior injuries
Straddle injury (fall, kick, cycle, etc.)	Fracture of pelvis (car accident, fall, crush)
Penetrating injury (gunshot, knife, etc.)	Penetrating injury (gunshot, stabbing, surgical intervention such as cystoscopy)
Instrumentation (catheters, cystoscopy, self-inflicted)	
Penile surgery (prosthesis placement or erosion)	
Sexual intercourse (penile fracture, urethral laceration)	

Medical surgical intervention

In both types of urethral trauma (anterior and posterior), the monitoring of urinary output is vital. In no case should a patient be catheterized until a continuous urethra can be seen on a urethrogram.

If surgical repair is needed, the urologist will site a suprapubic catheter. The surgeon is then free to perform a cystotomy and subsequently reconstruct the urethra, using a urethral catheter as a 'stent' by way of supporting the urethra during wound healing. This catheter will stay in place for up to 3 months, and will eventually be removed in a routine trial without catheter.

Some urologists are now opting for delayed repair of the ruptured urethra, performing a suprapubic catheter when the patient is injured and then operating 3 months later. This appears to have an associated lower risk of long-term complications, which include lower risk of impotence (10% risk) (Reilly 1995), incontinence and recurrent urethral strictures.

Nursing care

In all cases the nurse must observe vital signs and urinary output at regular intervals. If an intravenous infusion is present, the nurse must ensure that this is administered as prescribed. Analgesia should be given as indicated and as per prescription.

In post-urethroplasty patients standard postoperative care is required. Observations will include the care of and documentation of wound drainage. If the patient has a PCA, then this will require standard nursing care.

Before the patient is discharged home with his catheters in place, he should be educated regarding the care of them, and referred to a community nurse for support once he has gone home.

Urethral strictures

Urethral strictures are usually an acquired condition, and are most commonly found in men rather than women. This is due to the length of men's urethras, and their anatomical structure.

The cause of the stricture may be urethral manipulation during surgical procedures such as cystoscopy, long-term urinary catheterization or some form of trauma to the perineum in the form of a crush injury. In some cases, conditions such as neoplasms, warts or urethral polyps can also be causes of this condition (Carney et al. 1995).

When the urethra becomes injured, collagen and fibrous tissue will form at the point of injury, thus creating a narrowing of the urethra and reduction in elasticity (Figure 7.2). This has the effect of reducing the flow of urine.

Treatment of urethral strictures

The most common procedure used to treat urethral strictures is a direct visual urethrotomy (DVU), performed under general anaesthetic. During this procedure, the urologist will perform an incision through the full thickness of the scar tissue, which creates the stricture. This is done using a urethroscope. The urologist will then insert a Foley catheter (usually size 16 or 18 FG/Ch) in order to reduce bleeding and pain, and to keep the urethra patent (Carney et al. 1995).

The catheter will remain in place for a period up to 48 hours postoperatively, although this is usually decided on locally by individual consultant preference. In order to reduce the risk of recurrence

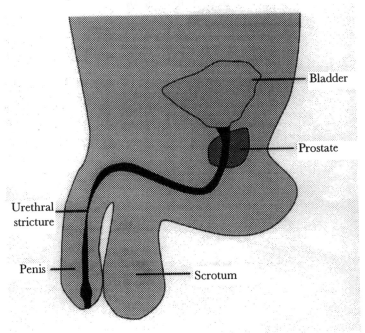

Figure 7.2 Urethral stricture.

of the stricture, the patient may be taught to perform CISC. The size of catheter and the frequency of performing this will be decided by the consultant. Incorrect size of catheter and incorrect frequency of the programme can cause further problems. Long-term use of CISC appears to be a possible cause of urethral trauma (Waller et al. 1997), and thus a contributing factor in urethral stricture formation.

In some cases, surgical reconstruction may be indicated, especially if dilation is required more frequently than 6-monthly intervals. It would also be appropriate if the size of the stricture is too great for DVU.

In this situation, a urethroplasty will be performed. This involves the excision of the stricture and rejoining the ends in an anastomosis. In some cases, a graft is needed to replace the excised urethra. As with the patient having a DVU, the patient will have a urethral catheter in place on return to the ward.

Decisions regarding the approach to treatment of the stricture will be taken on an individual basis by the consultant concerned with the case. Whichever treament is chosen, the success rate is high in the initial stages postoperatively. However, it now appears that urethral strictures will return in 30% of all cases, irrespective of the treatment option (Ragozzino et al. 1997).

Nursing care

The postoperative patient will require standard nursing care, including the recording and monitoring of vital signs, and urinary output through the catheter.

Once the catheter has been removed, a regular observation must be made regarding urinary output. The nurse must be vigilant in observing for acute retention of urine.

If the post-DVU patient is to perform self-catheterization, he must be taught this procedure before discharge. One of the most effective methods of patient education is use of visual aids such as computers or videos (Luker and Caress 1989), and this situation lends itself to use of videos. The patient should be shown a self-catheterization video, and then be instructed by the nurse in the process of CISC. Once competent, the patient will probably be allowed home on medical advice.

The nurse has a vital role to play in caring for individuals who have to perform CISC. Psychological support and encouragement are needed, because this procedure can be traumatic to some individuals – especially elderly men.

Meatal stricture

This is usually a congenital condition, although it can also be acquired as a result of infection or trauma (Gibbs 1995).

Patients with this condition will present with either reduced flow of urine, or it will be detected if a urinary catheter should be required.

Treatment of meatal strictures

The patient will need to be taught how to perform meatal dilatation using a plastic or glass dilator.

Nursing care

The nurse will be instrumental in the instruction and supervision of the patient performing meatal dilatation. The nurse's role includes psychological support and encouragement.

Urethral diverticula

There are two types of diverticula: primary diverticula, caused by congenital conditions (see Chapter 3); and secondary diverticula caused by infection, obstruction or instrumentation (Table 7.3). A secondary diverticulum could be caused by prostate abscesses or prolonged use of urinary catheters. In female patients, this could be caused by birth trauma or severe urethral infection.

Table 7.3 Urethral diverticula

Primary	Secondary
Congenital	Acquired
Mostly in men	In men and women
Possible incomplete urethral wall	Infection, instrumentation and obstruction possibly present
	Periurethral or prostate abscess possible cause
	Instrumentation of urethra
	Prolonged use of catheters
	Birth trauma

Urethral diverticula cause the urine to become trapped in a pouch in the muscle wall, and can obstruct the outflow of urine from the bladder. The trapped urine in the pouch is able to stagnate and become a focus for infection (Carney et al. 1995) (Figure 7.3).

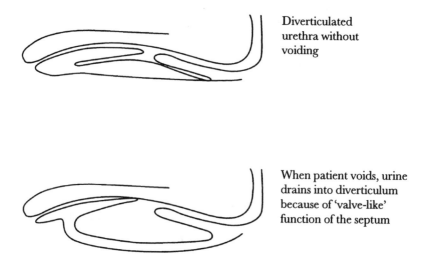

Diverticulated urethra without voiding

When patient voids, urine drains into diverticulum because of 'valve-like' function of the septum

Figure 7.3 Urethral diverticulum.

Treatment of secondary urethral diverticula

Urethral diverticulum needs to be confirmed using urethroscopy. If the diverticulum is large and causing problems, it will need transurethral drainage and resection.

Depending on consultant choice, there may be a decision to insert a suprapubic catheter. This will assist in healing the urethra by allowing time for the resection to heal.

Nursing care

The nurse will need to provide standard postoperative care, monitoring vital signs and urinary output.

If a suprapubic catheter is not present, the nurse will need to pay special attention to the voiding patient – observing for pain and possible signs of acute retention of urine.

Chapter 8
The testicle

IAN PEATE

Carcinoma of the testicle

Carcinoma of the testicle affects a relatively small number of the male population and those affected tend to be young men in their reproductive years. However, it is the most common malignancy in men aged between 15 and 35 years of age. Success rates are good when the malignancy is detected in the early stages. These success rates are above 90% and the term 'cure', as opposed to 'remission', is used confidently. However, 50% of men with testicular cancer are not diagnosed until the disease is in a more advanced stage (Rosella 1994). Table 8.1 demonstrates the relationship between age and rate of occurrence.

Table 8.1 Incidence rates of testicular cancer per million of the population (1983–85)

Age	Rate
0–4	7
5–14	1
15–24	34
25–34	89
35–44	72
45–54	32
55–64	18
65–75	15
75+	19

Source: Cancer Research Campaign (1991).

It has been noted that in some geographical areas the incidence of testicular cancer is higher than in other areas. Males from the Northern European regions have the highest incidence of testicular cancer per capita. In non-Caucasian populations the disease is less common. A genetic component may be responsible for the variations in white and black US men. It must be noted, however, that in non-Caucasian migrants there is no variation, hence it could tentatively be suggested that environmental influences may be the cause. Table 8.2 considers geographical variations.

Table 8.2 Geographical variation in cumulative incidence of testicular cancer among males aged 0–64 years

Low incidence (<0.2%)	Intermediate incidence (0.2–0.4%)	High incidence (>0.4%)
Finland	Australia	Denmark
India	Belgium	Hawaii (Whites)
Japan	Canada	New Zealand (Maoris)
Poland	Czechoslovakia	Ireland
Portugal	East Germany*	Luxembourg
Romania	European Community	Norway
Singapore	France	Switzerland
South America	Greece	West Germany*
Spain	Hungary	
USA (Blacks)	Iceland	
Yugoslavia*	Italy	
	Netherlands	
	New Zealand	
	Sweden	
	UK	
	USA (Whites)	

*Former.
Source: Cancer Research Campaign (1991).

Treatment of testicular cancer

There are three major treatment modalities associated with testicular cancer: chemotherapy, radiotherapy and surgical intervention. Before deciding which modality would be most appropriate for the patient, the nurse has a duty to explain the procedure in a language the patient understands, so that true informed consent can be achieved. The nurse should discuss with the patient the treatment, what it involves, the potential complications (long- and short-term) and the possible side effects.

Chemotherapy and radiotherapy

The administration of chemotherapy plays a major role in the treatment of testicular cancer. It plays an even more important role if there is evidence of metatastic spread. Treatment through a combined triple approach is commonly employed and when this is the case three drugs are used – bleomycin, etoposide and cisplatin (Neal and Hoskin 1997). They are usually administered over a 3-weekly period/cycle. Radiotherapy is also indicated in some cases and the degree or stage of the tumour is taken into account when deciding on the dose of radiotherapy.

Nursing issues

The use of chemotherapy and radiotherapy often renders the patient ill. The side effects of chemotherapy can be severe, ranging from pulmonary fibrosis to nausea and vomiting. The nurse has a vital role to play in ensuring that any side effects are detected in the early stages of treatment. Symptom control will promote well being and can encourage patients to continue with treatment. Sensitive and supportive measures are needed during this difficult period for both the patient and the family.

Surgical intervention

If surgical intervention is indicated then orchidectomy – either bilateral or unilateral – is required. More often than not unilateral orchidectomy is performed for testicular cancer (Fillingham and Douglas 1997). If a malignancy is detected, surgical exploration is undertaken and orchidectomy may proceed. The testicle is removed via an inguinal incision. As many of the cells of testicular cancer are malignant they are capable of being transmitted to healthy tissue, therefore testicular biopsy during the exploratory phase of surgery is contraindicated.

Nursing issues

The patient who undergoes orchidectomy will require general preoperative care. This type of surgery can have a profound effect on the patient's notion of body image. The testes are associated with manhood and the male's ability to produce viable sperm and thus father children. The patient's self-concept may be harmed and he may feel vulnerable in a societal setting and as a member of a family.

The man's ability to engage in sexual activities may be temporarily impeded. The skills the nurse brings with him or her will help to make this period of time more bearable for both the man and his partner. The use of sperm banks prior to treatment should be discussed with the patient in the event of long-term infertility. Often patients feel a sense of loss and may be pessimistic about the outcome of treatment. With continued support, a positive manner and encouragement, the nurse can help the patient come to terms with his illness.

The use of testicular prostheses for cosmetic effect may be appropriate. This will be performed 6 months after the original surgery, after discussion with the urology consultant.

Testicular self-examination and health promotion

Nursing issues

The main form of screening for testicular cancer in the population is through testicular self-examination (TSE). Early detection and prompt treatment will improve the patient's survival rate. Nurses, as health educators, have the ability to teach and promote TSE. The nurse, in a variety of care settings, should take every opportunity to encourage men to self-examine. Nurses provide holistic care and as such must also consider when is the appropriate time during the nurse–patient encounter to discuss TSE with men.

As testicular cancer affects the younger age range, nurses have a duty to target this particular age group. Carey et al. (1995) suggest that schools are an ideal place to begin to encourage young men to carry out TSE. It is well recognized that it is during childhood that particular health behaviours are often adopted. The behaviours adopted at this early age will impinge on adulthood. TSE is described in Table 8.3.

Orchitis

Acute orchitis is often caused by mumps in the adult. Laker (1994) states that orchitis as a result of infection by mumps occurs in 15–20% of adult males. Other viral infections, such as infectious mononucleosis and rubella, may also lead to orchitis. The result is a very painful swelling of the testes. Painful, swollen testes are also symptoms of other testicular conditions, such as torsion, therefore diagnosis of acute orchitis can be difficult. In the prepubescent boy the manifestation is torsion of the testes accompanied by an acute swelling of the testes.

Table 8.3 Testicular self-examination (TSE)

TSE takes only 3 minutes to perform. You should carry it out at monthly intervals, following the steps described below. This will enable early discovery of any abnormalities – diagnosis of testicular cancer usually begins with self-discovery. It is best to perform TSE after a warm shower or bath, when the scrotum is relaxed and the testicles are hanging lower from the body (it is normal for one testicle to hang lower than the other).

- Standing in front of a mirror visually inspect your scrotum for any signs of change – swelling or discoloration. Take your time and relax.
- Then place the pads of your index and middle finger of both your hands under one testicle and place the thumbs of both hands on top of the same testicle. Check one testicle at a time using both hands. Take your time and relax.
- Gently, squeeze your testicle and 'roll' it back and forth between your fingers and thumbs. Check the entire surface of the testicle while you do this.
- On the back of each testicle you will feel a small comma-like shape – the epididymis. This is normal. Check the epididymis for lumps. Towards the top of the epididymis you will feel the spermatic cord (vas deferens). Gently feel this for lumps and swellings.
- When you have done this to the first testicle move on to the other testicle, giving it the same examination. Take your time and relax.

What to look for
- Pain, swelling and hardness of the testes
- Conversely, a painless lump on the testicle
- Heaviness in the scrotum
- Aching in the lower abdomen or groin area
- An accumulation of fluid in the scrotal sac
- A change in the way the testicle feels.

If you discover any of the above you should seek urgent professional advice from your practice nurse or doctor. Remember, these symptoms do not necessarily indicate cancer, there may be other causes for the above symptoms

Bacterial infection of the testes may result in epididymo-orchitis. When the infection is the result of a urinary tract infection, the patient complains of a painful swelling of the epididymis, which often precedes the whole of the testicle becoming swollen. This swelling may be unilateral or bilateral.

Other causative organisms include the tuberculosis bacillus (TB). If TB is suspected, three early-morning urine specimens will be required for culture in the laboratory. TB is a difficult organism to culture, the urine specimens are cultured for the presence of acid fast bacilli (AFB).

Nursing issues

Orchitis is a very painful condition and the patient will require effective pain relief and the administration of prescribed antibiotic therapy. It is important that the patient rests, and the use of a scrotal support should be advocated to reduce the pain caused by swelling into the scrotal sac. In some instances the patient may be prescribed steroid therapy, which is thought to reduce the effects of testicular atrophy. If the patient complains of repeated attacks of orchitis it may be advisable to perform a vasectomy in an attempt to disassociate the epididymis from the urinary tract.

If TB has been isolated from the patient's urine, it is important that further investigations are undertaken to assess the extent of infection. Anti-TB medication will be prescribed and the nurse needs to instil into the patient the importance of completing the course of prescribed medication. This will also apply to patients who are prescribed antibiotic therapy. If steroids are used then patient education will include stressing the need to carry a steroid card and an explanation of why drug doses are to be reduced over a period of time.

The patient's occupation will need to be taken into account, and he must be discouraged from heavy lifting, as this has the potential to exacerbate the condition even further.

Other complications of orchitis may include the formation of abscesses. If this does occur, the abscess will need to be incised and drained under anaesthetic, and any necrotic tissue removed. In some cases orchidectomy may be needed, depending on the extent of necrosis; this is a rare but serious complication of orchitis.

As mentioned above, there is a danger that swelling of the testicle may lead to testicular necrosis. If this occurs it will result in reduced fertility or infertility, depending on the degree, and the patient may need to be counselled. Laker (1994) suggests that 50% of patients who suffer with orchitis will present with testicular necrosis, and if the condition is bilateral then there is a strong possibility that it will result in sterility.

Trauma

The testes may be injured during work (occupational injury), when playing sports, when engaging in vigorous sexual activity or during the use of sex toys. Nurses must be sensitive to the situation and how the trauma occurred if an in-depth patient history and assessment is to be made. Trauma can result in the formation of a haematocele – if there is a tear or a split within the tunica vaginalis blood leaks into the sac and causes swelling. The swelling, if left untreated, may constrict the testicle. This may result in atrophy, which can often lead to a malfunctioning testicle with possible infertility if spermatogenic function is damaged.

In all cases of testicular trauma ultrasound sonography is recommended, as an undiagnosed and therefore untreated testicular trauma can lead to loss of the testicle. In cases of severe testicular swelling and external bruising it is vital that scrotal exploration is undertaken, unless the results of the ultrasound demonstrate intact, 'normal' testes. If testicular injury is apparent the patient must be prepared for emergency surgery where exploration of the testicle will be undertaken, blood will be removed and the tunica vaginalis repaired. The procedure is usually carried out under general anaesthetic.

Nursing issues

As with acute orchitis, the patient should be encouraged to rest, be provided with scrotal support, given the prescribed analgesia and, above all, treated with sensitivity, as the nature of the injury may cause embarrassment. The patient will be advised to refrain from sexual intercourse for 2–3 weeks (this includes masturbation), and avoid sports and heavy lifting until the area has healed and he feels comfortable.

Testicular torsion

Testicular torsion can occur in males with descended or undescended testicles and more often occurs at puberty (Dawson and Whitfield 1997). When the testes and the epididymis rotate on the mesentery this is testicular torsion. If left untreated it can lead to obstruction of venous and, latterly, arterial drainage. Infarction of the testicle occurs and urgent treatment is needed. Laker (1994) suggests that if the blood supply is reduced for longer than 6 hours then complete infarction is likely to occur.

The patient will complain of sudden, acute pain in the testicle, and referred inguinal or abdominal pain may be experienced. The testicle will be painful to touch and may be oedematous. Diagnosis is made on clinical history and examination. The diagnosis of epididymo-orchitis, strangulated hernia or testicular tumour may also be considered. If there is any doubt about the diagnosis it should be presumed to be testicular torsion until proven otherwise.

Nursing issues

Exploration of the scrotum is needed, and the patient must be prepared for emergency surgery. In some instances the torsion can be corrected by untwisting the testicle. It is rotated first one way and then the other; a distinct click will be felt and the patient will feel immediate relief. Prior to rotation the patient will need pain relief. The torsion is corrected under general anaesthetic and the viability of the testicle is assessed. If it is infarcted then orchidectomy is needed. If the testicle is viable it is fixed to the excised edge of the tunica vaginalis and the inner layer of the scrotal skin. If the other testicle is found to be equally mobile it too is secured at the same time. This procedure is called orchidopexy.

Infertility

Infertility affects approximately 10% of all couples (Laker 1994). In nearly one third of cases the infertility is due to a low or absent sperm count or impotence. Female-related problems account for another third, and the final third are said to be related to problems existing in both partners.

The production of viable sperm – spermatogenesis – is a complex process and involves many stages. Spermatozoa are produced in the testes and transported through the vas deferens to the seminal vesicles, where other substances are added to produce viable, motile spermatozoa. Physically, the male partner needs to be able to maintain an erection to facilitate penetration and also have the ability to ejaculate. If anything interferes with the male's ability to carry out any or all of the above he will be deemed infertile.

The production of sperm begins in the seminiferous tubules, which are surrounded by Leydig cells. The Leydig cells produce testosterone. When follicle-stimulating hormone (FSH) is released by the pituitary gland, spermatogenesis begins.

During this process, the basilar membrane of the seminiferous tubules, which contains two types of cells – spermatogonium and Sertoli cells – undergoes change, and these cells become primary and secondary spermatocytes, and eventually spermatids. The spermatids grow into spermatozoa, which are released into the seminiferous tubules via the lumen and then sent to the epididymis via the ductal system. The sperms at the tail end of the epididymis (as opposed to the head end) are said to be more fertile.

Spermatozoa are sensitive to heat, and are produced at a temperature a few degrees lower than body temperature. It is the dartos muscle in the scrotum that will relax or contract in response to changes in environmental temperature to maintain testicular homeothermy, by either raising the testicles closer to the abdomen or relaxing them. The testes of an individual with untreated cryptorchidism remain at body temperature, which will inhibit spermatozoa production, rendering him infertile.

Immature and non-motile spermatozoa mature in the epididymis, where they are stored until required. They leave the epididymis via the ejaculatory duct. When ejaculation occurs the seminal vesicles contract and seminal fluid is forced into the common ejaculatory duct, then on to the prostatic urethra. At the point of ejaculation the prostatic gland contracts, the bladder neck muscles contract and the internal urethral orifice is closed. Rhythmic contractions transport the semen along the length of the erect penis. The semen is finally deposited into the female's vagina.

In addition to the above there are other factors that need to be considered. Men who had one or both testicles undescended at birth will have a lower semen quality than men whose testicles were normally descended at birth. The production of viable spermatozoa can also be affected if a man has experienced testicular torsion and a degree of infarction has occurred, rendering the testicle less able to produce motile, viable sperms. Mumps orchitis after puberty can also affect the production of viable sperms, as can the use (or abuse) of certain drugs, including salazopirine, caffeine, nicotine, alcohol and marijuana.

Some surgical procedures can impair fertility. Post-bladder neck incision, there is a 40% chance that a man will experience retrograde ejaculation (Dawson and Whitfield 1997). The risk of infertility is even higher after transurethral prostatectomy. Testicular blood supply and the vas deferens may be damaged when inguinal herniorrhaphy is performed. Dawson and Whitfield (1997) suggest that interruption of the sympathetic nervous system may occur during resection of retroperitoneal lymph nodes; this interruption results in failure to ejaculate.

To assess the patient fully, a general physical examination is carried out, noting the presence or absence of secondary sexual characteristics. Any abnormalities, such as hepatomegaly or gynaecomastia, may suggest that the patient is suffering from hypogonadism or hormonal imbalance. During the physical examination the man should be asked to lie down and his testes examined visually and physically. There may be evidence of varicocele. In 2% of infertile men the vas deferens is reported to be absent (Dawson and Whitfield 1997), this therefore needs to be located and palpated.

Investigations of infertility in men

One of the first investigations will be analysis of the seminal fluid. However, it must be noted that it is inappropriate to judge a man's fertility on this analysis alone; other factors must also be taken into account. The interpretation of the results will direct the form of treatment. To obtain an adequate semen specimen it is imperative that the correct procedure is used. The man should abstain from ejaculation for at least 3–5 days before producing the masturbated specimen, and it is vital that the specimen is analysed within 1–2 hours of production. The characteristics of normal semen are given in Table 8.4.

Table 8.4 Normal characteristics of semen

- Semen volume >1.5 ml
- Sperm concentration >20 million per ml
- More than 70% of spermatozoa should be motile
- Motile grade >2: where 0 = no movement and 4 = excellent forward movement
- More than 60% of sperms should have normal morphology
- Fructose should be present in the semen

Source: Adapted from Dawson and Whitfield (1997).

Hormonal evaluation may be carried out. If testicular sperm production is altered due to lack of FSH, the levels of FSH and luteinizing hormone (LH) will be elevated (Figure 8.1) (McCance and Huether 1994). If azoospermia occurs when the concentration of FSH is normal, testicular biopsy and a vasogram are needed to determine if the azoospermia is a result of testicular failure or vasal obstruction.

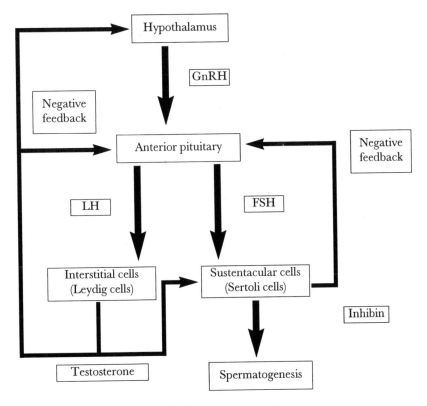

Figure 8.1 Hormones associated with spermatogenesis.

If the pituitary gland fails to produce FSH or LH, there will be a reduction in the amount of testosterone produced by the Leydig cells in the testes. Hence, a variety of factors may be responsible for infertility in males.

When the cause of the infertility points to impotence, further investigations are required (see Chapter 10). Again, an in-depth patient history/assessment is needed and the initial assessment will include the points listed in Table 8.5.

Nursing issues

Whatever the cause and treatment decided upon, the nurse has the ability to ensure that the patient and his partner receive high-quality care. Infertility should be regarded as a joint problem. Infertility clinics have as a fundamental tenet the ability to offer couples counselling. When the couple have been given information about prognosis and treatment options, the nurse must provide support to both parties. The decisions arrived at are based on individual needs, and counselling should aim to assist both individuals. Much of the nursing care will be based on the psychological aspects of infertility and the nurse must bear in mind that the patient and his partner may be experiencing a great deal of emotional stress. The help formulated need to take this into account.

Table 8.5 Contents of initial assessment

- An in-depth sexual history
- Is there any evidence of impotence occurring during periods of elevated stress, e.g. financial worries, marital or work-related problems?
- Is the impotence insidious in origin?
- Failure to maintain erections may point to venous leakage

Vasectomy

The ultimate goal of vasectomy is to arrest the flow of spermatozoa through the vas deferens. The procedure is usually conducted under local anaesthetic on a day-surgery basis. An incision is made in the scrotum, the vas deferens are located and a section is removed. To prevent the vas from rejuvenating and rejoining, the cut ends are turned back on themselves and ligated (tied off).

Vasectomy has little if any bearing on a man's ability or desire to have sexual intercourse, although in some instances a man may encounter psychosexual problems. There is a slight possibility that the ligated ends of vas deferens may rejuvenate and rejoin, thus viable sperm may appear in the vas deferens, and it is vital that both parties are made aware of this.

Post-vasectomy, a man will be able to resume normal sexual activity as soon as he feels comfortable, but some form of contraception must still be used until his semen has been analysed and demonstrates azoospermia. This may take up to 6 weeks post-ligation.

Nursing issues

Nurses must be aware that in certain institutions the consent form for vasectomy may need to be signed by both the patient and his partner. It needs to be stressed to both the patient and his partner that reversal of vasectomy is not always successful, indeed the success rate is poor. The notion of informed consent for both parties cannot be overemphasized.

In 1% of patients who undergo vasectomy there is haematoma formation (Laker 1994; Simpson 1998). The haematoma may be large enough to warrant surgical intervention (Laker 1994). To reduce the risk of haematoma formation the patient should be encouraged to rest for 1–2 hours post-vasectomy. A well-fitting scrotal support will promote comfort and reduce haematoma formation. It is normal for a degree of bruising to occur and this may be accompanied by a mild degree of pain and discomfort.

To prevent infection, the patient should be encouraged to shower daily and keep the area clean and dry. If infection is present it is usually caused by the patient's own infected semen, and antibiotic therapy may be prescribed.

It is important that the nurse provides the patient with information that promotes a safe discharge from the day surgery unit. He should be told to contact his GP or the day surgery unit's telephone helpline if he has any problems, and an appointment must be made for further semen analysis 8 weeks after surgery. The patient must be told how to collect the semen sample.

The scrotal support should be worn until the bruising has subsided or when the patient feels comfortable without it. Sexual activity can be resumed as soon as the patient feels comfortable and nurse must reiterate the need to use contraceptive devices until the semen analysis demonstrates azoospermia. He can return to work as soon as he feels able to – usually within a week. Driving should be avoided for 1–2 weeks.

Vasovasostomy

This procedure aims to reverse the effects of vasectomy. Laker (1994) suggests that there is an 80–90% chance that spermatozoa will appear in the ejaculate of men post-vasovasostomy. There is a 40–70% possibility that the partners of these men will become pregnant. It is important that men who request vasovasostomy are aware of the lower and upper bracket success rates if they are to make a truly informed decision preoperatively. The success rate is confounded further; the rate of success is dependent on (among other things) the time interval between having the vasectomy and the vasovasostomy. The greater the time lapse the less chance of success.

The procedure is more intricate than the original vasectomy and the nurse has a duty to fully inform the man about the impending operative procedure. Vasovasostomy requires a general anaesthetic and may take up to 2 hours to perform (Fillingham and Douglas 1997). The nurse must make this clear, as the man may have the mistaken belief that this procedure will be similar to a vasectomy. The nurse must conduct an in-depth nursing assessment of the patient and bear in mind his ability to withstand a general anaesthetic.

Usually, a lower abdominal or scrotal incision is made and the aim then is the anastomosis of the cut ends of the vas deferens. Postoperatively, when assessing the patient's analgesic requirements, the nurse must be able to differentiate between the type and severity of pain caused by vasectomy and vasovasostomy, the latter being much more painful. The effects of general anaesthesia may cause more problems than those of local anaesthesia, and the wound may be more prone to infection than the vasectomy wound. There is also an increased risk of haematoma formation.

Nursing issues

The patient should be encouraged to rest in bed on the day of the operation and in some instances on the second postoperative day also. Strenuous exercise should be avoided, as should unnecessary lifting. It often takes 2 days to recover from the procedure. Prior to discharge the nurse needs to ensure that the patient is fit for discharge and able to cope at home.

Hydrocele

Hydrocele is a structural disorder of the testes and scrotum. It is a collection of fluid in the tunica vaginalis, and can be caused by a tumour, injury or infection. It can present either unilaterally or bilaterally. There are three main types of hydrocele:

- primary
- congenital
- secondary.

In primary hydrocele the patient is often middle-aged and the cause is idiopathic. In congenital hydrocele the processus vaginalis has failed to close or closure is late, allowing peritoneal fluid to enter the cavity. In most such cases, spontaneous closure of the processus vaginalis occurs and the hydrocele disappears. Secondary hydrocele occurs as a result of injury to the testicle or as a response to inflammation.

The patient rarely complains of pain as a result of the fluid collection, but the size and weight of the enlarged scrotum may cause discomfort, anxiety and embarrassment. The nurse's approach to the situation must be sensitive.

The usual mode of treatment is aspiration of the hydrocele under local anaesthetic, on a day-surgery basis. The testicle is transilluminated so that the practitioner can identify the position of the testes. A trochar and cannula are inserted and the fluid is drawn off. The nurse must physically and psychologically support the patient during the procedure. If the fluid aspirated is blood-stained (taking into account that the blood may result from traumatic insertion of trochar and cannula), further examination of the scrotal contents may be needed. An ultrasound scan may be requested to rule out malignancy.

Often, however, the hydrocele reoccurs and may require intermittent tapping. If this is the case the patient may be offered the opportunity to undergo surgical treatment to excise the hydrocele sac. This procedure is called hydrocelectomy.

Hydrocelectomy is performed under general anaesthesia. An incision is made in the scrotal sac, the fluid is drained off and a series of sutures are inserted to effectively close the potential space and prevent the possibility of further fluid accumulation. This procedure can be very painful and the patient will need appropriate analgesia postoperatively. A large haematoma usually appears post-surgery, and the nurse should provide the patient with a scrotal support to promote comfort and assist in the reduction of oedema. To reduce postoperative anxiety, the patient should be told beforehand that swelling is likely to occur, but that this is quite normal and may take a few weeks to subside. The nurse should note the degree of haematoma formation, as haemorrhage can often be concealed in the scrotal sac. If the surgeon has left a drain in situ this will need to be managed appropriately. An ice pack can be gently applied to the area to further reduce the oedema. The patient will require individual information regarding a return to his normal lifestyle.

Acknowledgement

I would like to acknowledge the help given by Mrs Frances Cohen.

Chapter 9
Gender reassignment

Jeanne Beckett and Janet Hall

Gender reassignment is the term ascribed to the process by which a transsexual client is able to approximate the anatomic structures and characteristics of their identified psychological gender.

Transsexualism is the name given to the condition in which the individual feels that their gender, as ascribed by anatomical sexing at birth, is at odds with their identified psychological gender. Medically defined as a gender identity disorder, that is gender dysphoria. The term transsexual is reported by Leiter et al. (1993) as originating in the late 1940s with the work of Caudwell. The concept of the condition described as gender dysphoria evolved from the research undertaken by Harry Benjamin in the 1960s (Benjamin 1966). He identified the condition from his observations of patients under his care who presented with conflicts of gender. Although this work can be called descriptive, it is recognized as being some of the earliest psychological research into the area of gender identity disorders.

Gender identity is recognized as being pivotal to all aspects of an individual's life. Walters and Ross (1986 p 2) analyse this concept further and divide it up into the following components:

- Psychological
  - gender identity (sense of being male or female)
  - social sex role (masculinity or femininity)
  - public sex role (living or dressing as male or female)
  - sexual orientation (homosexual, heterosexual, asexual)
  - sex of rearing (brought up as male or female).

127

- Biological
  - genetic (presence or absence of Y chromosome)
  - gonadal (histological structure of ovary or testis)
  - hormonal function (circulating hormones, end-organ sensitivity)
  - internal genital morphology (presence or absence of male or female internal structures)
  - external genital morphology (presence or absence of male or female external genitalia)
  - secondary sexual characteristics (body hair, breasts, fat distribution)

The client presenting for gender reassignment is principally concerned with the concept of psychological versus anatomical gender. However, as can be seen from the breakdown of gender identity, the concept of gender is multifaceted and complex. Therefore the care pathway for clients presenting with gender dysphoria is equally as complex.

Care pathway

For the purpose of this chapter the care pathway refers to the treatment of individuals suffering from gender identity disorders and does not include the treatment of children suffering from congenital adrenal hypoplasia, androgen insensitivity syndrome, hermaphroditism or any congenital chromasomal abnormality (although the authors do recognize that there is a similarity in some of the medical and surgical treatments involved).

The care pathway, as already stated, is complex and multifaceted. However, for this chapter it has been simplified by being divided into four principal areas, that is psychological, endocrinological, surgical and societal. The latter, although not a medically recognized treatment area, is necessary for the client to successfully integrate into the social gender of their identified psychological gender, arguably the principal aim of any treatment plan.

It is estimated that 1 in 15 000 people in the UK is transsexual; of these only 25% will be female to male. Due to the covert nature of the condition, statistics are limited to the number of individuals who declare themselves and/or present for treatment.

Not all clients suffering from gender dysphoria choose to travel the full length of the care pathway, culminating in surgery. Some may be satisfied with psychological and endocrinological treatment. This is particularly common among female to male transsexuals due, perhaps, to the experimental stage of female to male surgery and to the fact that the outcome of hormone therapy for the female to male transsexual tends to produce a societally acceptable male. In addition, it can perhaps be argued that historically it has been regarded as acceptable for a female to aspire to be male, but a man wanting to be seen as female has been an object of derision.

Psychological

The initial entry to a gender reassignment programme is by reference to a qualified psychiatrist or psychologist who will perform an in-depth psychological profile. The aim of this is to exclude an organic psychological illness, such as schizophrenia, and to assess the transsexual's suitability for gender reassignment.

The clients are usually assessed according to the criteria evolved from the work of Benjamin (1966). These criteria have been updated over time (Benjamin 1981), and include the following:

- Lifelong cross-gender identification.
- An inability to adapt to, or function in, assigned biological gender.
- Compliance with a medically defined programme of psychotherapy.
- Possession of a convincing appearance of the chosen gender.
- Ability to successfully live and work in the cross-gender role.
- Demonstration of stability, that is long-term relationship and employment.
- Ability to demonstrate an understanding of the limits of gender reassignment and a realistic expectation acknowledging that reassignment can only approximate the physical characteristic of their chosen gender and, at present, has nothing to do with the procreation of children.
- Completion of at least one year of medically supervised hormonal treatment. The latter condition does not apply in the UK as it is usual for the client to attend for psychological assessment before hormone treatment is commenced.

Endocrinological

The endocrinological (hormone) treatment comprises the administration of appropriate hormones, which will enable the individual to develop a more acceptable physical appearance appropriating that of their psychological gender. This is a gradual progression that mimics to some degree the transitional role of puberty. However, unlike puberty, this is not a natural event and, like any other individual embarking on a programme of hormone therapy, transsexuals need to undergo a detailed physical screening including ECG, fasting blood lipids, full blood count, urea and electrolytes, liver function tests, blood glucose and chest X-ray. The aim is to identify clients who may be at risk of the complications of such therapy and for whom the administration of hormone therapy could be life-threatening. That is, clients suffering from, among other things, severe hypertension, ischaemic heart disease, cerebrovascular disease, hepatic dysfunction, impaired renal function, poorly controlled diabetes and hypertriglyceridaemia.

It is important that the client is made aware of any complication risks before embarking on hormone therapy.

Male to female

The aim of oestrogen therapy is to suppress testicular activity, demasculinize and oestrogenize.

Medications currently in use are:

- Premarin 2.5 mg three times a day
- Ethinyloestradiol 50 mcg twice a day
- Androcur 50 mg twice a day.

These medications are given orally and have the side effects of any oral oestrogen, namely nausea and vomiting, hypertension, oedema, increased tendency to blood clotting leading to thrombosis and embolism. In addition there is the long-term risk of liver failure.

The effects of the hormone therapy are gradual and include:

- a reduction of libido and subsequently morning erections, the latter tending to correlate with a reduction in the serum testosterone levels
- a shrinking of the testes
- a softening and slower growth of facial hair
- an improvement in facial acne
- a gradual cessation of scalp hair loss

- a reduction in muscle mass
- a gradual change in the distribution of body fat to give a more feminine contour, and also nipple tenderness and some increase in breast size. However, the latter varies from individual to individual and can be a disappointment to some clients.

Female to male

The aim of the androgen therapy is to masculinize.

Medications currently in use are:

- Sustanon 250 mg
- Primoteston Depot 250–500 mg.

These medications are given by intramuscular injections at 2-weekly intervals. The side effects include hypertension, oedema, increased erythropoiesis due to the direct stimulating effect of the bone marrow causing increased red blood cell mass, liver enzyme abnormalities and hyperlipidaemia, which can increase the risk of cardiac disease.

The results of the therapy are again gradual and include an increase in libido, cessation of menstruation, an increase in body and facial hair and in some cases some thinning of the scalp hair, a change in pitch (deepening) of the voice, a change in the distribution of body fat and an increase in muscle mass. Unfortunately the reduction in the breast tissue is minimal and there will be an identifiable need for surgical intervention in the future.

The changes in the genitalia vary from individual to individual and some clients experience a degree of enlargement of the clitoris, which may make them suitable candidates for metaidioplasty in the future.

Surgery

Gender reassignment surgery for the transsexual whether male–female or female–male is a complex issue. For the male–female transsexual it involves mammoplasty, augmentation mammoplasty, castration, orchidectomy, penectomy, and plastic surgery to feminize facial features and reduce the size of the crichoid cartilage. For the female–male transsexual this involves mastectomy, hysterectomy, salpingectomy, oophorectomy and vaginectomy. In addition, both sexes desire external genitalia that are aesthetically acceptable and functional for sexual purposes and allow micturition to be performed in the gender-biased socially acceptable position. However, for the urological nurse the area which is most relevant to his or her practice is that of genital surgery and, therefore, other aspects of surgery such as mastectomy are not addressed in this chapter.

Male to female

The genital surgery for the male–female transsexual consists of: penectomy, preserving the glans and its blood supply; construction of labia and vagina; and the creation and placement of the neo-urinary meatus. Techniques for this surgery are improving over time and it is now possible to offer clients aesthetically acceptable genitalia that are sexually and mechanically functional.

Notification of date for surgery

A patient information booklet needs to be sent out with the notification of the client's date for surgery. Research identifies that this should contain information about surgery including: realistic expectations of outcome; instructions about stopping hormone treatment completely by 3 weeks prior to surgery; details of any side effects that may occur; reassurance that no long-term damage will be done, i.e. they will not revert to being male; general information about the ward and hospital; and guidance about suitable clothing for wearing while an inpatient. Much of this information appears to be common sense but for some transsexual clients who are isolated in their new condition, basic information can save a lot of postoperative distress and disruptive behaviour.

Preadmission clinic

Anaesthetic and medical assessment, will be carried out:

- Bloods are taken for urea and electrolyte estimation, full blood count, liver function tests, group and cross-matching blood for two units.
- Mid-stream urine is obtained for routine testing and culture sensitivity.

- ECG and chest X-ray are performed when medically indicated.
- Flow rate and bladder scan are performed to provide a baseline of bladder function.

The client will have an appointment with the urology nurse specialist/counsellor to enable her to voice any matters that may be worrying her and to reinforce information given in the preadmission booklet. This offers an ideal time for the client to visit with her partner, explore their expectations and to discuss realistic outcomes of the surgery.

Nursing assessment within the nursing model currently in use can be commenced at this time to identify specific needs, such as does the client wear a wig, or have any facial hair growth that necessitates shaving, and to reiterate the fact that the client will be required to remain on bed rest for 4 days. Anecdotal evidence has shown that this inactivity has been a problem for some clients in the past. This is also the ideal time to begin discharge planning.

A ward visit and introduction to the nurses who will care for the client should also be undertaken.

Preoperative care

Admission to the ward is the day prior to surgery. The primary nurse having access to the pre-admission notes can discuss further any anxieties the client may have.

A visit is arranged with the pain control sister to discuss postoperative pain control and with the physiotherapist to discuss and practise postoperative exercises. A sachet of Klean-Prep is given to empty the bowel, not only to prevent faecal contamination intraoperatively but, as postoperatively the patient will have a pressure dressing covering the perineal wound including the rectum, defecation is undesirable. Fluids only are given overnight.

On the day of surgery the client is prepared for theatre as per hospital protocol having been given nil orally for 4 hours prior to estimated time of surgery. Ted stockings are applied as a preventative measure for deep vein thrombosis. Pubic shaving is undertaken in theatre.

Surgical procedure

Epidural anaesthesia is used, as well as a general anaesthetic, in order to reduce bleeding in what is a very vascular area.

The patient is placed in the lithotomy position, the perineal and suprapubic area shaved and draped:

1   A midline perineal incision is made up to the urethra, the testes are identified, dissected up to the inguinal ring, double ligated and removed. Both are then sent for histology.
2   The skin of the penis is then circumcised at the corona and dissected off the shaft.
3   The neurovascular bundle is isolated and with the glans dissected off the corpora. The corpora is then removed.
4   To allow positioning of the urethra and vagina to approximate the anatomy of the female, the anterior abdominal wall, skin and fat only, is mobilized and pulled down and fixed to the pubic bone with nylon sutures tied over serbo pads. A drain is then inserted.
5   The urethra is then dissected off the rectum up to and behind the bladder, divided and catheterized.
6   The penile skin is oversewn to form the neovagina. A plane is made by blunt dissection between the urethra, anterior and rectum, posterior, approximately two fingers' width. The pelvic floor muscles are divided with cutting diathermy and the inverted penile skin is placed in the gap.
7   The glans is trimmed, placed and sutured on to the anterior part of the neovagina to form the clitoris. The urethra is inserted into the anterior part of the neovagina in a position that will enable the patient to sit down to pass urine without spraying the floor. It is then recatheterized, spatulated and partially oversewn in an attempt to prevent stenosis occurring. A gauze pack is then inserted into the neovagina.
8   The scrotal skin is trimmed with inverted Y and V flaps to form the labia and a pressure dressing is applies.

Postoperative care

The client will be safely returned to the ward, conscious and pain-free. IV fluids are administered for the first 24–48 hours. IV antibiotics are given for 3 days to prevent infection and heparin daily until discharge as a further measure to prevent deep vein thrombosis.

The client will have a wound drain, urethral catheter and vaginal pack. The perineal wound will be encased in a pressure dressing. The urethral catheter must be secured to the client's leg at all times to prevent pain or traction damage to the neourethra. The pain control of choice is epidural analgesia or PCA, both of which are titrated according to the individual client's pain score.

Vital sign observations are measured 1–4 hourly according to level of stability.

The immediate complication that can occur is hypovolaemic shock due to bleeding from the neovagina, neourethra or wound. Treatment is aimed at stopping the bleeding. The pressure is removed and bleeding points sutured, either under local anaesthetic or in theatre, and the pressure dressing is replaced. Blood transfusion is prescribed according to haemoglobin estimation and measurable blood loss.

Bedrest is maintained for 4 days, during which the client will need to be provided with facilities to undertake any cosmetic activities she feels necessary, including for some clients removal of facial hair growth by shaving.

Oral fluids are commenced when the client is able to tolerate them, as is a light diet.

The vaginal pack is removed on the fourth day and the client is taught to dilate her neovagina with a size 1 or 2 dilator, leaving the dilator in situ for 20 minutes. It is important that the client understands that if the vagina is to remain patent this is a lifetime commitment. The dilators are now manufactured and are available in various sizes, size 1 being the smallest. At the same time the neoclitoris is inspected for viability, as are the neolabia. The neolabia at this stage are likely to be bruised and swollen. The client is then taken for a bath and encouraged to sit out of bed for a period.

By the fifth day the client is encouraged to walk about, ensuring that the urethral catheter is secured and the neourethra is protected from tension trauma.

Emotionally during the immediate postoperative period many clients are elated but on around the fifth day many clients experience a period of depression rather similar to the 'baby blues' experienced by postpartum females. Unfortunately this can lead to disruptive behaviour by some clients and can be avoided if clients are forewarned that this may occur and are cared for by empathic nurses.

The sorbo-rings and associate sutures are removed on the sixth day, and hormonal therapy is resumed on the seventh day. The urethral catheter is removed on the eighth day and a catheter specimen of urine is obtained and sent for microscopy to exclude any catheter-introduced infection. The client needs to be advised how to position herself when passing urine, as she may experience some initial spraying which can be distressing.

The aim of the nursing care is to enable the client to pass safely through the surgical process of gender reassignment. Gelder et al. (1989) suggest that although there is no characteristic type of personality associated with gender dysphoria, some transsexuals can be self-centred, demanding and attention-seeking, and can be particularly difficult to treat. Anecdotal evidence from practice has found this to be true, therefore, in addition to the technical care, there is necessarily a high input of psychological care.

Long-term complications

- Closure or shortening of the neovagina due to the client not continuing daily dilation. Unfortunately this can only be treated by vaginal reconstruction either by skin graft or by major reconstruction using a portion of the large bowel.
- Prolapse of the vagina, treated by surgical repair.
- Urethral stenosis, needing surgical dilation followed by regular dilation.
- Overgrowth of the neoclitoris or labia, both of which can be trimmed to improve the cosmetic appearance.
- Rectal fistula is a major, but fortunately rare, complication that can occur during the operative procedure when the plane is being made between the bowel and the bladder to accommodate the neovagina. Repair of such fistula involves further major surgery.
- Lack of ongoing psychological support has been reported as resulting in mental breakdown, severe depressive illness or suicide.

Optimum results

The optimum result of male to female gender reassignment is a psychologically stable individual living in her chosen gender with the option to be sexually active if she so desires.

Female to male

Surgical techniques within the area of genital gender reassignment for the female–male transsexual compared with techniques for male–female gender reassignment are still in the experimental stage. This is due to the problem of creating a male phallus (phalloplasty) that is aesthetically acceptable; is capable of sustaining an erection capable of penetrative sexual intercourse; and also of providing an organ of micturition that will enable the 'new man' to micturate in a standing position. Included in the genital surgery is the need for the construction of an aesthetic bifid scrotum in which testicular prostheses can be inserted.

In the past, the literature has suggested that vaginectomy and mastectomy should be among the precursors to the more complicated surgery of phalloplasty. However, a current literature search reveals that the vagina and breasts of the female–male transsexual may have a place in the construction of a viable phallus.

Hage (1995), from Amsterdam, describes a technique called metaidioplasty that, in some cases, can be used to surgically enhance the clitoris that has been enlarged by hormone therapy to produce a phallus that is functional and aesthetically acceptable to the client. To do this, he uses a caudally based pedicled flap raised from the anterior wall of the vagina and constructs a bifid scrotum using labial tissue, into which testicular prostheses can be inserted. According to the literature his surgical techniques results in a small penis that is aesthetically acceptable and enables the client to micturate standing up. However, although it retains sensation it is not large enough for vaginal penetration.

Safak et al. (1996), in Turkey, describe their first attempt at penile construction using a lateral thoracic flap from breast tissue that would usually have been removed at mastectomy. The graft was transferred microsurgically to the genital area, with the clitoris being incorporated into the base of the neophallus. The entire technique was complex and necessitated various procedures over a period of 8 weeks in total. Early indications, however, were that the technique resulted in a good-sized, aesthetically acceptable penis through which the patient could micturate standing up. No indication was given in the literature about whether the function was sufficient for penetrative sex.

A pedicle skin graft from the lower abdominal wall is still one of the most common methods of creation of a neophallus, although the advent of microsurgery has resulted in the use of a radial forearm flap gaining popularity. It is suggested that with the insertion of a penile prosthesis these methods can offer the client a cosmetically acceptable phallus through which he can void urine standing up and which is firm enough for vaginal penetration.

Nursing care

The preadmission and preoperative psychological care are as for the male to female transsexual, with particular emphasis on ensuring that the client has realistic expectations of the surgery and understands that he will need to undergo a series of surgical procedures. It is important to emphasize that he will have some residual scarring in the donor area. This can be a particular problem following a radial forearm graft.

Preparation for theatre is as before.

Postoperative care

Bedrest is maintained for 4–7 days as per surgeon's instructions. The graft is protected from accidental damage by a padded dressing, and the site is inspected at designated intervals.

A urethral catheter is left in situ to act as a stent for the neourethra. A suprapubic catheter is used to drain the bladder. These are left in situ according to the individual surgeon's treatment plan.

The donor area is dressed with a non-adherent dressing, which is not removed until the tenth day, unless there are signs of infection, by which time most of the area should be healed.

IV antibiotics are administered for 3–5 days. Heparin is given until discharge to prevent deep vein thrombosis.

Complications

- Poor circulation to the graft resulting in loss of some or all of the grafted skin.
- Infection in the grafted skin, resulting in the above.
- Lack of sensation in the grafted skin.
- Stenosis of the neourethra.
- Poor healing of the donor area, requiring skin grafting.
- Unacceptable, to the client, scarring to the donor area.
- Deep vein thrombosis, pulmonary embolism.
- Hirsutism of the neophallus due to changes in the skin of the donor area, brought about by the administration of testosterone. This is a cosmetic problem and can be dealt with by the judicious use of proprietary hair-removing creams.

The outcomes of phalloplasty are variable and depend on the skill and experience of the surgeon involved.

Societal

The societal aspects of gender dysphoria are of paramount importance if the client is to integrate successfully into their psychological gender group. These aspects include both outward appearance and lifestyle documentation, marriage, divorce, pension and employment rights, and imprisonment.

Appearance

The current tendency for intersex clothing and behaviour has made it easier for the female–male transsexuals to dress gender-appropriately and to integrate successfully into their chosen societal gender group. However, for the male–female transsexuals the road is still beset with problems. It is not merely a question of dressing as a female but of learning the speech patterns and mannerisms acquired by females over time. Various voluntary agencies now run courses that aim to address these problems and teach the appropriate social skills.

Nursing intervention

Nurses may be required to teach social behavioural skills to clients within their care so that they may fit into the ward or clinic environment. This may involve discussing appropriate nightwear, underwear or other clothing for use in the mixed environment of the ward. Anecdotal evidence suggests that poor or little advice in this area can result in the client being isolated and the victim of derision by other patients. Clients that need this help should be identified during the preadmission nursing assessment.

Lifestyle documentation

Birth certificate

Under the umbrella of English law, although gender reassignment is irreversible, the entry on the birth certificate recording sex at birth cannot be changed to show the postoperative sex. Under English law, sex and gender are synonymous and are decided at birth on the basis of biology, that is the external appearance of the genitalia. The Registrar of Births and Deaths, however, has the power to change the entry if there is a proven factual error, such as can occur in the case of ambiguous genitalia when the individual's sex can be scientifically proven. Because of the anathema attached to birth registration of the transsexual, his/her death must be registered in his/her designated sex, a matter that can cause intense distress for family and friends.

Marriage

The ongoing effect of not being able to change the entry on the transsexual's birth certificate is that a male–female transsexual cannot marry a male and a female–male cannot marry a female. However, this exposes an anomaly in law in which a postoperative transsexual does not have to divorce his/her current partner, effectively a marriage between persons now of the same sex (Rogers 1993). Various applications for a change in the law have been made to the European Court of Human Rights. Harris et al. (1995) identified the problem as arising from Article 12: 'The right to marry and found a family which refers to the traditional marriage between persons of the opposite biological sex and primarily concerned with protecting the concept of the family and the procreation of children.' If this was to be taken to its extreme logical outcome, then all persons who did not wish to or could not procreate would be unable to marry. This rule is confined to English law and transsexuals who wish to marry can go abroad to do so on the understanding that on their return their marriage is not recognized within the UK.

Divorce and pension rights

Divorce can only be arrived at through the same legal channels as for non-transsexuals, therefore the recent changes in the law regarding pension rights in which divorcees have a claim on their partner's pension are not affected (Denning 1996).

Retirement pensions

Under current legislation in the UK, a postoperative transsexual is still registered as a member of his/her preoperative sex, therefore a male–female transsexual would not be entitled to claim state retirement pension until the age of 65 and conversely a female–male transsexual would be eligible at the age of 60.

Imprisonment

At the present time a transsexual can be incarcerated in a prison appropriate to their registered gender; however, the practice is currently under review.

Employment

The Equal Pay Act and the Sexual Discrimination Act 1975 has given protection in law for transsexuals (Denning 1996). However, during the transition period of gender reassignment a transsexual in the public eye may chose to move sideways to a less public area. This should be a personal choice and, in law, gender reassignment should not be seen as a barrier to promotion and any employment change should be with the transsexual's consent.

Everyday documentation

Under English law, a transsexual can change his/her name to one more appropriate to their psychological gender. This is done by deed poll or statutory declaration and relates to medical card, income tax, passport, driving licence, bank accounts, utility bills, examination records and insurance documents.

With regard to life insurance, the picture is clouded by the normal gender differences. Therefore it is necessary for the individual transsexual to declare his/her change in status.

Transsexuals' sexuality and the care team

The sexual orientation of the transsexual client is no different from the general population in that they may be heterosexual, lesbian, asexual or occasionally homosexual. However, some of the concatenations may be difficult for members of the care team to understand. For example a male to female postoperative transsexual may be in a lesbian relationship with another female. The RCN gives guidelines for the care of the gay client but does not approach the topic of the transsexual client and the sexual ambiguities that may be exposed.

In addition, the age range of clients currently presenting for surgery (male to female) is 20 to 60+. Many of them may have been married in their former lives and have fathered children. This is common in the older age group, in their attempt to appear more masculine, because prior to the change in the law in 1967 it was unacceptable for a man to declare himself homosexual, let alone declare that he felt he was a female.

Experience has shown that these clients are acutely aware of any incongruence or empathy among the care team and on a practical level this can be a catalyst for disruptive behaviour. It is essential for units offering gender reassignment surgery to provide an equally high standard of care for their own team, with the setting up of counselling services and regular discussion groups to give the team time to be themselves and to explore their own feelings with regard to this particular client group. This can only result in personal growth and an increased understanding and improvement in patient care.

Conclusion

The emphasis within the NHS of treatment according to 'need' as opposed to 'want' means the case for treatment for the transsexual patient can be a controversial one, particularly as due to the covert nature of the condition the long-term outcomes are not able to be validated by research. All that can be said is that anecdotal evidence shows that without the opportunity for treatment many of these clients would not survive and that with treatment many are able to integrate successfully into the culture of their psychological gender. Thus they are enabled to live 'normal' lives.

Chapter 10
Erectile dysfunction

PHILIP DOWNEY

Erectile dysfunction (or impotence as it is more commonly known) is an issue that appears to affect two million men in the UK (Holmes 1998a). However, this figure may well be underestimated, as witnessed by the enormous press and public interest shown since the launch of new oral medication during the latter months of 1998. The true figure is yet to be determined.

Erectile dysfunction is defined as the inability to maintain or achieve an erection for satisfactory sexual performance (and this is used in its broadest context) (Ashford 1998). This condition can have a profound impact on the man and his partner – creating additional mental anguish for both parties.

The causes of erectile dysfunction are numerous, but are usually separated into two categories, namely psychological or physical.

Psychological causes

The processes associated with erection are dependent on psychological input. This means that there may be inhibition of erection by a psychological disturbance (Ashford 1998). The brain, therefore, can affect the erectile mechanism by sending out inhibitory neural signals through the spinal cord, and through the systemic release of catecholamines (Holmes 1998a).

This type of impotence can be caused by depression, problems within a relationship, and anxiety. It is also common for this to be self-perpetuating, because further sexual episodes are overshadowed by the fear of failure that develops after a previously unsuccessful sexual episode (Holmes 1998a).

Psychologically caused erectile dysfunction usually presents with rapid onset. Nocturnal and early morning erections usually still occur. It is the most common type of impotence in young men (Holmes 1998a).

Treatment of psychologically caused impotence

A full medical and sexual history should be taken with patience, sufficient time and privacy, along with a physical examination. Communication skills and an open non-judgemental attitude are essential (Ashford 1998).

Treatment for this kind of impotence can be either simple or complicated. The simple solution may well be to encourage the man and his partner to take advantage of an early morning erection and engage in sexual activity on waking up (therefore breaking the cycle of fear of failure).

Lifestyle changes may be appropriate. Advice may be needed concerning smoking, drinking or recreational drug usage. Stress, if this is a factor, may need to be tackled with relaxation therapy. In some cases, men may gain an improvement in quality of erection if they perform regular pelvic floor exercises (Ashford 1998).

However, not all cases are so simple. In some cases, both men with this kind of impotence and their partners are most likely to benefit from psychosexual counselling – since sexual dysfunction is frequently inseparable from relationship problems (Ashford 1998).

Physical causes

Approximately 80% of men who present with erectile dysfunction will have a physical cause for their condition (Slag et al. 1983). It can be the result of vascular, neurological or endocrine disorders.

Neurological abnormalities

Erectile dysfunction created by neurological causes tend to follow spinal injury or pelvic trauma (including surgery). It is possible, in some cases, that this type of impotence is a sign of diabetic neuropathy or multiple sclerosis.

Vascular abnormalities

These include problems with the blood flow in or out of the penis. Insufficient blood supply can be seen in men who smoke, or who suffer with hypertension, diabetes, or other cardiovascular or peripheral vascular disease. Pelvic surgery may result in damage to the penile blood supply.

If the blood supply out of the penis is the cause of the dysfunction, this is classed as a venous leak or veno-occlusive dysfunction.

Endocrine causes

The role of testosterone in connection with erectile dysfunction is as yet unclear. However, low levels of serum testosterone appear to create a loss of libido and, on some occasions, erectile dysfunction (Lue 1991).

Disorders of the pituitary and thyroid glands may also have an impact on erectile dysfunction.

Treatment options of physical causes

Vacuum constriction device

A cylinder is placed over the well-lubricated penis and a seal is created at the pubic area. A pump is activated, thus creating an erection. This then causes blood to be drawn into the penis, thus creating an erection. When the erection appears to be sufficient, an elastic ring is pulled from the canister on to the base of the penis, and the pump is removed.

An erection will persist for the duration of time that the ring is in situ, with a recommendation that the ring is removed after approximately 30 minutes (Ashford 1998).

Advantages of this device include the fact that it is one of the safest and least expensive methods available. Most men will achieve an erection with the device. However, success is largely dependent on adequate training (Gilbert and Gingell 1992).

Disadvantages include the fact that the vacuum-created erection is liable to feel cold, and can appear mottled in colour. It is also important to remember that the penis is only erect from the elasticated ring, and it is possible for the man to experience 'penile fracture' as a result (see Chapter 7). The man may also feel discomfort from the ring. Overall, most complaints seem to be around the issue of spontaneity, and the need to interrupt their sexual activity to use the vacuum pump (Ashford 1998).

Injection therapy

The main drugs of choice until recently, were injections into the corpus cavernosum. Papaverine and phentolamine are two currently unlicensed drugs that have been very effective in the treatment of men with impotence, and have been developed since the early 1980s. The licensed drugs for injection include alprostadil, and this is perhaps the most commonly used product.

The dose of alprostadil (like all of the others) is carefully calculated, in order to give the man an erection for a period of approximately one hour. The patient is taught how to inject the drug using a fine-bore needle. It is vital that at this stage the patient is informed of the possible side effects – most notably priapism.

Advantages of this method of treatment include response rate (approximately 70% of men will respond to this treatment) (Ashford 1998).

Once the man is used to self-injection, the use of this therapy can be quite discreet, and some men have reported that spontaneous erections will occur after long-term use of the therapy.

Disadvantages include priapism, if the dose is incorrect, or the patient does not realize the dangers of prolonged erection. Manual dexterity is also an issue. Some men may not be able to manipulate the syringe effectively, and some individuals have a fear of needles. Lack of spontaneity is also an issue.

All these issues need to be addressed when deciding on the most appropriate treatment.

Oral medication

Unprecedented coverage about the condition of erectile dysfunction was demonstrated during 1998, when the media heralded the arrival in the UK of the 'wonder drug' sildenafil – commonly known by the trade name Viagra – as the cure-all, treat-everyone drug for impotence. Widespread usage in the USA was reported in the press, along with the side effects of cardiac arrest, etc. The true success rate of this drug has yet to be discovered in the UK where it has only been licensed since September 1998.

An alternative to sildenafil is the unlicensed drug yohimbine. This is an alkaloid that is said to have some aphrodisiac properties. Success rate is not confirmed, but it appears to enjoy a good success rate in people with psychologically originated impotence.

Transurethral prostaglandin therapy

This is a new approach to treating erectile dysfunction. To date, this treatment, which involves delivering a small pellet of prostaglandin into the urethra, appears to be encouraging (Gingell 1998). It has been available since the beginning of 1998, under the name of MUSE (medicated urethral system for erection).

The man is taught that he should urinate prior to insertion of the pellet using an applicator. MUSE is quick and easy to use, and studies have shown that up to 80% of the prostaglandin is absorbed within 10 minutes of administering the drug, creating a significant increase in blood supply sufficient to achieve erection. It appears to be effective, regardless of age or cause of erectile dysfunction.

In some cases, men have reported penile pain. Some have reported dizziness, hypotension and urethral trauma. No episodes of priapism have been reported. Overall, it would appear that MUSE is a safe and effective treatment choice (Gingell 1998).

Penile implants

These are used for men who have failed with all other treatments; in most cases these individuals will have insufficient arterial flow. Implants involve the removal of the existing erectile tissue within the corpora. Preoperative counselling regarding the possible postoperative complications is essential.

There are two types of prosthesis available for men with impotence, namely semi-rigid or inflatable.

Semi-rigid prostheses
This is by far the simplest device, comprising two separate rods which are inserted under general anaesthetic into the corpora. They can be bent either up for sexual intercourse, or down for normal use.

Cosmetically, these devices are limited. They can be difficult to conceal when the penis is in the 'flaccid' state, and they neither

improve girth nor length measurements of the penis when it is used
in sexual intercourse (Holmes 1998b).

Nursing issues. Following this operation the patient will have a
perineal wound. Nursing issues surrounding this type of prosthesis
include the observation of vital signs on a regular basis. The wound
should be checked for signs of infection. Wound healing may be
delayed in the diabetic patient. Urinary output also needs to be
observed in case the patient goes into urinary retention (thus requiring the insertion of a suprapubic catheter in this instance).

Inflatable prostheses
This comprises two cylinders, a pump and a reservoir. It yields the
most effective cosmetic result. The pump for this is located within
the scrotum, and inflation of the device works on the principles of
hydraulics. There is a deactivation button to facilitate deflation of
the prosthesis, thus allowing the prosthesis to subside.

Satisfaction rates are higher for the man's partner in comparison
with the semi-rigid prosthesis, although again the prosthesis will not
increase the length or girth of the erect penis (Holmes 1998b).

The man needs to be able to demonstrate reasonable manual
dexterity to use this device successfully. Because the prosthesis is
mechanical, there will be a greater risk of mechanical failure.

Nursing issues. The patient will have a suprapubic wound, and in
most cases will return to the ward with the penis strapped upwards
on to the lower abdomen in an attempt to reduce the risk of swelling.
He will probably be catheterized and the nurse needs to pay attention to the vital signs and urinary output of the patient.

The device will be activated in clinic. This is done approximately
6 weeks after insertion in theatre, therefore allowing the wounds to
heal adequately.

Prostheses that have been ill-fitted can lead to erosion of the
device through the skin, or cause a drooping of the glans. Erosion
may appear months after the fitting of the device (Holmes 1998b).

Venous leak surgery

In some cases, the ligation of penile veins will provide a possible solution to their erectile dysfunction. It involves the stripping of the
dorsal vein and ligation of the visible veins that drain the corpora.

Results of this approach are poor, with a less than 50% success
rate. It has also been argued that the same results would be achieved

by using a constricting band around the base of the penis (like those used in the vacuum device therapy) (Holmes 1998b).

Nursing issues in erectile dysfunction

Nurses need to be aware of the fact that erectile dysfunction affects not only the man but also his partner. It can also have a profound effect on his self-image and therefore may well cause problems with social interaction and his workplace. It has been suggested that in 21% of cases, erectile dysfunction has been a contributory factor in the breakdown of relationships. It is also reported that men with this condition recorded low self-esteem, embarrassment and feelings of inadequacy or rejection (Ashford 1998).

If nurses are aware of these facts, they will be able to work with these men and their partners in a sympathetic and constructive manner.

Chapter 11
Catheter design and selection

PENNY WESTBROOK

Introduction

A tenth of all hospital patients in the UK will have an indwelling catheter inserted (Getliffe 1996a), while 4% of patients receiving community nursing will be catheterized (Winson 1997). Catheters have developed considerably from the primitive hollow leaves of onion plants coated with lacquer, first used in China in 100 BC, to the sophisticated materials of the present day (Bloom et al. 1994).

Catheterization can range from short-term, just a few hours, to long-term, from months to even years (Winn 1996; Winson 1997). Demographic changes and an emphasis on care in the community mean that catheterization has become an increasingly necessary form of treatment (Getliffe 1993; Kohler-Ockmore and Feneley 1996). It is an invasive procedure carrying many risks and therefore it should aim to increase the patient's quality of life, and not create further problems and complications (Kennedy and Brocklehurst 1982; Willis 1995a).

This chapter discusses why patients are catheterized and probes the process of catheter selection. The scope of materials used in the manufacture of catheters is highlighted, stressing their suitability for each patient's requirements. The range of drainage systems available is also addressed.

The physical and psychological well being of patients is vitally important, and thus must be borne in mind by nurses, who remain the patients' advocates. The decision to catheterize should be a joint one between the patient, carer and health professional (Rigby 1998). Catheterization should not be considered as permanent, but reviewed on a regular basis (Getliffe 1993). Rigby (1998) also suggests that nurses should be involved in all stages of catheterization; from the initial joint decision, to the actual insertion and the long-term management of the catheter.

Nurses should also be providing evidence-based practice, which means keeping up to date with new developments and technologies evolving from recent innovations and research (Willis 1995a; Winn 1996; Rigby 1998), which results in a rapidly widening catheter market.

Indications for catheterization

1. Acute or chronic retention of urine, where outflow of urine is impaired by urethral stricture, benign prostatic hyperplasia, bladder neck obstruction or disease (e.g. prostate cancer) (Willis 1995a).
2. Untreatable urinary incontinence when all alternatives such as continence aids have proved unsuccessful or impossible (Getliffe 1996a; Willis 1995a; Woollons 1996). Research suggests that of all patients catheterized in hospital or in the community, almost half would have been catheterized due to urinary incontinence (Kennedy and Brocklehurst 1982; Kohler-Ockmore and Feneley 1996).
3. Accurate monitoring of urine output during acute illness (Getliffe 1996a; Winn 1996).
4. During severe or terminal illness catheterization will improve patient quality of life (Rigby 1998).
5. Neuropathic bladder, where there is difficulty in completely emptying the bladder (e.g. spinal injury, multiple sclerosis) (Getliffe 1996a).
6. As an aid to surgery, either before or following, to allow access for the drainage of clots or debris (Willis 1995a; Winn 1996).
7. Urological diagnosis, e.g. urodynamics (Winn 1996).
8. Instillation of cytotoxic therapy, e.g. to treat papillary cancer (Willis 1995a).
9. Bladder irrigation, for bladder lavage following surgery to drain blood clots (Rigby 1998).

Catheter selection

Often it is the nurse who influences the medical staff's decision to catheterize in both hospital and community patients (Willis 1995a; Winson 1997), and it is the nurse who also selects the most appropriate catheter for the procedure (Willis 1995a).

There is a wide variety of catheters on the market, and the number is constantly increasing as a result of the developments in materials and coatings technology, which are aimed at the production of a catheter compatible with the human body (Bull et al. 1991). Nurses therefore need to be aware of recent research developments within this rapidly changing field (Willis 1995a).

Nurses should consider the following criteria when selecting the most appropriate type of catheter for either indwelling or intermittent catheterization (Willis 1995b; Woollons 1996):

- minimal complications
- ease of insertion and removal
- comfortable in situ
- can remain in situ for maximum recommended time
- tissue compatibility.

The decision to catheterize and the type of catheter should ultimately be based on the assessment of the patient's needs and made in agreement with the patient. The following points should be considered (Hodges 1997; Rigby 1998; Willis 1995a):

- how long the catheter is to stay in place
- what the patient's urine is like
- male or female patient
- the size of balloon required
- the patient's general health
- bladder capacity
- bowel habit (as constipation should be avoided)
- dexterity – aids are available.
- comprehension/mental ability, the nurse may need to gain support from family members or carers
- sexual activity.

Once the catheter is in situ the patient should be continuously monitored and evaluated as the patient's catheter needs may change over time, from an indwelling to an intermittent catheter (Hodges 1997; Willis 1995a).

Material selection

The most appropriate catheter will be the one that will stay in situ for the maximum recommended time, is comfortable for the patient and has the least number of complications.

There are four types of catheter material available:

- latex
- latex-coated
- all silicone/all hydrogel
- PVC (plastic).

They range from short-term to long-term application (Willis 1995a). Nurses must be familiar with the correct use of each catheter and the associated complications, and be up to date with recent research findings.

Latex

Latex, made from natural rubber, is the most common type of material used for short-term catheters (7–10 days) (Willis 1995a). Although resilient, pliable and flexible, it has a number of disadvantages, including latex allergy and an unsmooth surface, which increases the risk of urethral trauma leading to urethritis and even strictures (Laurent 1998). Consequently, the use of uncoated latex is diminishing and no longer recommended (Getliffe 1996a; Willis 1995a; Woollons 1996). Furthermore latex absorbs water causing the catheter to swell, reducing the internal lumen and increasing the external diameter. It becomes encrusted during short-term use as encrustations are produced as a result of increased alkalinity in the urine and this leads to the formation of crystalline deposits on the catheter surface (Kohler-Ockmore 1991; Wilde 1997; Willis 1995a; Winn 1998; Woodward 1997). Research has found that over half of all patients with indwelling catheters are prone to blockage due to encrustation (Winn 1998), and patients can be classified as either 'blockers' or 'non-blockers' (Kohler-Ockmore 1991). These blockages result from bacterial biofilms and encrustations (Lowthian 1998). Latex also hardens with age and therefore the use-by date must be strictly adhered to prevent the catheter hardening within the body (Lowthian 1998).

To comply with toxicity level standards, new, improved latex-coated catheters are now being manufactured (Cox 1990; Woodward 1997) using Teflon, silicone and hydrogel to coat the catheter surface. These special coatings aim to reduce the incidence of encrustations by limiting bacterial biofilm adhesion. However, despite the manufacturers' claims, these special catheter coatings cannot prevent blockages completely (Lowthian 1998).

Latex coatings

This category of catheter is suitable for short-term to medium-term use.

Teflon (PTFE)-coated latex

Used for 3–4 weeks, Teflon (PTFE)-coated latex is smoother than plain latex, which helps to prevent encrustation and irritation (Laurent 1998; Willis 1995a). The smoother surface also aids insertion and removal, and absorption of water is reduced due to the Teflon coating. This type of catheter is more cost-effective than silicone-coated or hydrogel-coated catheters (Woodward 1997).

Silicone / silicone elastomer-coated latex

For mid-term use, up to 6 weeks. The impregnation with silicone oil means that the catheter is easier to insert, causing less friction and tissue irritation (Cox 1990; Laurent 1998). However, the oil is thought to permeate out of the latex during the first few hours in situ (Cox 1990). As with PTFE, water absorption and consequent swelling is reduced (Laurent 1998). It also has a zero toxicity rating and is the most commonly used catheter (Bull et al. 1991; Woodward 1997), although evidence suggests that this catheter is more likely to result in bypassing than the hydrogel-coated catheter (Winn 1998).

Hydrogel-coated latex

Recommended for long-term use, up to 12 weeks. This catheter possesses similar properties to the silicone-coated catheter (Woollons 1996). It is also the catheter most compatible with human tissue and is therefore the most comfortable (Willis 1995a). Polymers absorb water to form a soft gel, which makes the catheter surface slippery and easier to insert. It is thought to be more resistant to encrustation and bacterial colonization than other types of catheter (Cox 1990; Laurent 1998). However, research evidence suggests the contrary. Morris et al. (1997) found that the hydrogel-coated catheter is quicker to block than the all-silicone catheter. The hydrogel-coated catheter is associated with less bypassing and leakage (Bull 1991; Woollons 1996). However, it is more expensive than silicone-coated and Teflon-coated catheters and should therefore be used only if it is to remain in situ for the recommended time. It is not suitable for patients with a known tendency towards encrustation.

Although these coatings exhibit obvious benefits over the use of pure latex, the additive does diffuse out over time and can ultimately lead to tissue irritation and reaction. Consequently, they do not fully protect against latex allergy (Woodward 1997).

100% hydrogel

Hydrogel resembles living tissue and thus this type of catheter, suitable for long-term use up to 3 months, is easier to insert than other catheters (Willis 1995a). It has a reduced risk of urethral damage and is associated with reduced episodes of bypassing, and is therefore the patients' preferred catheter choice. This catheter, like 100% silicone, is expensive and for them to be cost effective it is important to keep these catheters in for the full recommended time. Therefore a history of any previous catheterization is important in assessing whether a patient is prone to encrustations and blockages, and establishing a catheter life for that patient.

100% silicone

This is the most expensive type of catheter, but is the one least likely to cause allergies and tissue inflammation (Lowthian 1998; Winn and Thompson 1998; Woollons 1996). Like the hydrogel catheter, to be cost-effective, it must be used in the long term for up to 3 months. It is a thin-walled catheter with a large internal diameter drainage lumen (Laurent 1998). It is associated with reduced encrustation (Woodward 1997), although bacteria will eventually adhere to it (Winn 1996). This is supported by research evidence, with all silicone catheters being found less likely to block over a 14-day period, when compared with coated latex (Morris et al. 1997; Winn 1998).

Unfortunately research has shown that the balloon is susceptible to water loss once in situ, and although this is a slow process (Lowthian 1998; Wilde 1997; Winn 1998), it can result in the premature replacement of the catheter (Barnes and Malone-Lee 1986). Therefore it should be evaluated every 2 weeks while in situ and water lost from the balloon replaced as necessary.

Polyvinyl chloride (PVC)

The cheapest type of catheter material used is plastic, usually polyvinyl chloride (PVC). It is recommended for short-term use (7–10 days) in postoperative drainage or for intermittent catheterization. As the plastic is stiffer, providing greater rigidity, the catheter walls can be made thinner. This not only makes it easier to introduce but also allows a better flow of urine (Laurent 1998; Willis 1995a). Although the plastic does soften at body temperature it still remains hard, inflexible and uncomfortable in situ (Willis 1995a), and it is prone to crack and quick to develop encrustations (Laurent 1998).

Catheter types

There are three main categories of catheter:

- ballooned urethral catheter
- urethral catheter (without balloon)
- suprapubic.

Ballooned urethral catheter

This is also known as the self-retaining or indwelling catheter, of which the 'standard two-way Foley catheter' is the most frequently used long-term urethral and suprapubic catheter (Willis 1995a; Woollons 1996) (Figure 11.1).

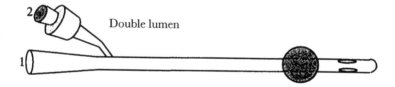

Figure 11.1 Ballooned urethral catheter: two-way Foley. 1: Channel for urine flow; 2: Channel for balloon inflation.

The two-way Foley catheter has a double lumen with one channel for urine flow and another channel for balloon inflation using sterile water (Willis 1995a; Woollons 1996). The other type of catheter is the three-way irrigating catheter, with one channel for urine flow, a second for balloon inflation and a third for continuous or intermittent irrigating fluid (Willis 1995a) (Figure 11.2).

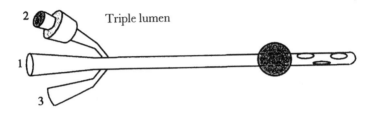

Figure 11.2 Ballooned urethral catheter: three-way Foley. 1: Channel for urine flow; 2: Channel for balloon inflation; 3: Channel for irrigation.

The balloon is positioned near the tip of the catheter but beneath the drainage eyes, and once inflated it sits at the sensitive base of the bladder. The size of the balloon is important, and although most balloons can accommodate as much as 200 ml of sterile water they must be filled according to the manufacturer's guidelines. This cannot be stressed enough, since underfilling or overfilling can distort the shape of the balloon and thus affect the position of the catheter, which can result in erosion damage to the bladder mucosa (Britton and Wright 1996; Wilde 1997; Woollons 1996).

In the community, it is an advantage to use prefilled balloon catheters with reservoirs of sterile water. After insertion a plastic clip is removed to release the water and fill the balloon. This eliminates the use of syringes and sterile water ampoules (Getliffe 1993; Woollons 1996).

Balloon size

Although modern balloons are thin-walled to reduce irritation to the bladder, it is still important to use the smallest balloon size possible, usually 5–10 ml capacity. In some instances, however, e.g. post prostatectomy, a 30 ml balloon will be indicated (Willis 1995a). Too large a balloon can result in spasms, bypassing and ulceration of the bladder or urethral walls (Hodges 1997; Willis 1996, 1998). It can also lead to infection, as the eyes of the catheter will sit too high in the bladder, leaving a greater residual volume of urine and a reservoir for infection (Getliffe 1996a). Research demonstrates that in many instances catheters with balloon capacities of 30 ml are chosen despite this being contraindicated (Crow et al. 1988).

Urethral catheter (without balloon)

This catheter type has only one channel for drainage and is not intended to remain in situ for long periods of time. It is applicable for use in the following situations (Willis 1995a):

- obtaining pathology specimens
- bladder emptying before surgery or urodynamics studies
- treating urethral strictures
- to instil drugs inside the bladder
- intermittent self-catheterization to manage incontinence.

Made from rigid PVC to aid insertion, the most popular type is the Nelaton catheter (Figure 11.3) (Cowan 1997), which has two drainage eyes at the tip and a funnel end. This is of benefit to patients with poor eyesight ensuring that the correct end is inserted (Winn and Thompson 1998).

Nelaton 12CH

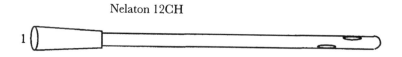

Figure 11.3 Intermittent catheter: Nelaton. 1: Channel for urine flow.

The Gibbon catheter is another non-ballooned catheter which is used in patients with enlarged prostates and urethral strictures. It is externally fixed to the penis with adhesive tape and is available in small sizes.

Other available catheters have hydrophilic coatings, which require no additional lubricant. After immersing in water, the surface becomes slippery, making it easier to insert. However, these tend to be more expensive and are for single-use only (Winn and Thompson 1998).

Clean intermittent catheters

Intermittent catheters are used in:

- spinal nerve damage, e.g. multiple sclerosis
- poorly functioning detrusor muscle
- overflow incontinence due to enlarged prostate
- urethral strictures requiring self-dilatation (Hodges 1997; Willis 1995a; Winn and Thompson 1998).

Clean intermittent catheterization can be performed by a patient or carer and is becoming an increasingly popular way of managing continence problems (Willis 1995a), although it is not used extensively due to a lack of awareness (Cowan 1997). It has several advantages over the use of the self-retaining urethral catheter, including an increased quality of life, greater independence and dignity, and a reduction in the incidence of urinary tract infections (Bakke et al. 1997).

Clean intermittent catheterization needs to be performed several times a day, either in the short term or long term, and therefore requires a high degree of motivation, physical dexterity and mental capability. Consequently, nurses must carefully assess each patient's physical and mental ability as well as their motivation before instigating a teaching programme (Willis 1996).

Suprapubic catheters

The suprapubic catheter is an alternative to an indwelling urethral catheter and is often used for patients with urethral trauma (Peate 1997). The catheter is introduced into the bladder surgically, under local anaesthetic, through the abdomen wall. Initial insertion is always by a doctor and should be used only in cases where the patient has an easily palpable bladder, e.g. acute or chronic retention of urine (Hodges 1997; Lowthian 1998; Peate 1997; Willis 1995a), and never in people with a known bladder tumour.

There are three basic types of suprapubic catheter. The first is a combination type Foley catheter with balloon and flanges, which are sutured to the abdomen. The second type has wing-style attachments that hold it in place, while the third is a self-retaining balloon-type catheter (Laurent 1998).

The suprapubic catheter is available in sizes 6–16 (French gauge), and can be changed through the original track without further anaesthetic, provided the new catheter is introduced immediately to prevent the track from closing. This procedure can be performed by nurses and carers with adequate training, according to local hospital or community policy (Willis 1995a). However, we would recommend that medical staff perform the first catheter change because of the risk of the track closing over. Nurses should perform only the second and subsequent changes.

Some clinical nurse specialists are now undertaking training to allow them to carry out the initial insertion of suprapubic catheters, in accordance with the UKCC Scope of Professional Practice (Peate 1997; Rigby 1998; UKCC 1992).

The suprapubic catheter has several advantages over urethral catheters, including greater comfort, patient dignity, fewer infections and the option for patients to have sexual intercourse as normal (Hodges 1997; Peate 1997). The disadvantages include potential leakage, altered body image, paucity of nursing research and the requirement of a medical practitioner at the initial insertion (Peate 1997).

Although often used following urethral trauma, other indications for use include those patients unable to tolerate a urethral catheter, some wheelchair-bound patients and patients recovering from gynaecological surgery (Peate 1997). The insertion of a suprapubic catheter involves a surgical wound and thus a strict aseptic technique must be adhered to during the management of the catheter. Dressings and tapes should only be used when absolutely necessary, and then minimally, as they can provide a potential site for infection (Peate 1997).

Catheter size

Catheter size is referred to as either 'French gauge' (FG) or 'Charrière gauge' (Ch), describing the size in terms of the external diameter of the catheter. Most catheters are available in sizes 8–24 FG/Ch, where '8' refers to the smallest paediatric catheter size and '24' the largest, often used for heavy haematuria, usually following urological surgery. Confusion can arise when choosing the most appropriate catheter size for each patient, and nurses must be aware that the larger catheter size does not imply larger drainage eyes.

The smallest catheter size that allows adequate drainage should be used in all patients (Hodges 1997; Woollons 1996), unless there is debris present in the form of mucus or heavy haematuria with clots.

Usually sizes 12–16 FG/Ch are most appropriate in adult cases. Women may be better able to tolerate the use of the larger size 16 FG catheter, which is likely to cause problems in men due to the presence of tight curves in the male urethra (Lowthian 1998). Too large a catheter can result in bypassing, due to urethral irritation; patient discomfort; and even pressure necrosis, resulting in urethral strictures (Hodges 1997; Willis 1996).

Catheter length

British standard regulations stipulate that all catheters must conform to a minimum length: 38 cm in men, 22 cm in women and 22 cm in paediatric patients (Laurent 1998). The length of the female catheter takes into account the shorter length of the female urethra, which not only respects the patient's dignity, but also prevents accidental trauma or blockage due to kinking, pulling or looping of the extra catheter tubing (Willis 1995a; Winn and Thompson 1998; Woollons 1996). The exception involves obese female patients, where the longer, male catheter is more appropriate (Winn and Thompson 1998). The manufacturer Bard has designed the female 'Conformo-cath', which not only considers the length of the female urethra, but also the shape. Unfortunately, it is not available on prescription (Woollons 1996). Despite literature supporting the use of the appropriate catheter length, research evidence in one study highlighted that the female catheter was used in only five out of 165 female patients investigated (Crow et al. 1998).

Specialist catheters

There are a variety of specialist catheters available on the market for specific uses. The Tiemann tipped catheter (Figure 11.4) with its curved tip is often used for patients with prostatic hyperplasia or an obstructed urethra (Willis 1995a). The Coudé tip catheter, similar to the Tiemann, has one, two or three drainage eyes situated in the curved tip (Britton and Wright 1996).

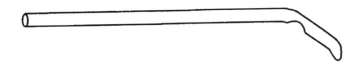

Figure 11.4 Tiemann catheter.

The Whistle tipped catheter (Figure 11.5) is mainly used postoperatively for drainage of large clots and debris. This is facilitated by the large drainage area supplied by the lateral eye in the tip and the eyes above the balloon (Britton and Wright 1996).

The Roberts tip catheter (Figure 11.6) also facilitates greater drainage, with eyes above and below the balloon, and it is therefore suitable where residual volume is a problem (Britton and Wright 1996).

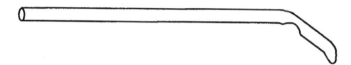

Figure 11.5 Whistle catheter.

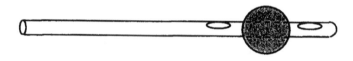

Figure 11.6 Roberts catheter.

Drainage bags

To promote patient dignity and comfort, drainage bags should be selected according to the individual's preference, especially if they are for long-term use, when it is also preferable for the patient to try a variety of bags before selecting the most appropriate one (Roe et al. 1988). This is important, considering the number of bags that are available, ranging from a 2-litre bag with measuring device, which is often seen in a hospital environment, to a smaller leg bag, which is attached to either the thigh or lower leg (Getliffe 1996a; Roe et al. 1988).

Attachment of a leg bag is a debatable issue. It is argued that strapping the catheter to the leg could cause traction and restrict drainage (Pomfret 1991; Winn 1998). However, most literature advocates securing the catheter to the leg, thus ensuring support and preventing sphincter damage (Winn 1996). Applying adhesive tape to secure the catheter to the leg is not supported, as it can cause damage to the special catheter coatings that are often used (Winn 1998).

In an attempt to delay bacterial access to the lumen of the catheter (Lowthian 1998) the closed urinary drainage system (CUDS) (Figure 11.7) should be maintained. Disconnection of the catheter and drainage tubing should be avoided (Lowthian 1998), and it is recommended that the CUDS remains intact for 5–7 days (Willis 1995b; Winson 1997). If the system is broken a new drainage system should be attached (Willis 1995b). However, evidence suggests that changing drainage systems frequently increases the rate of infection (Winson 1997).

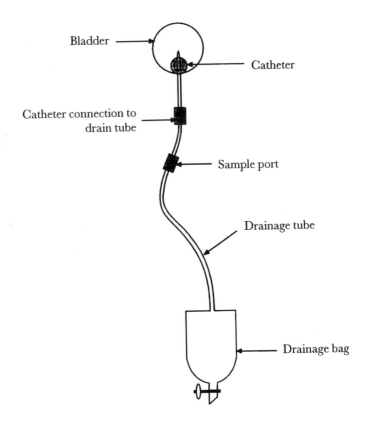

Figure 11.7 Drainage system: leg bag and catheter valve.

Overnight bags can be attached to leg bags without breaking the CUDS, and can be reused if washed and dried within the patient's own home, where there is a low risk of cross-infection. In hospitals, however, disposable bags should be used (Roe et al. 1988; Winson 1997).

The use of catheter valves as an alternative to leg bags has increased in popularity in recent years (Fader et al. 1997), and research evidence suggests that it is preferred among patients (German et al. 1997). The catheter valve is attached to the catheter outlet and thus urine is stored in the bladder and not in the drainage bag. Releasing the valve allows intermittent drainage of the bladder. However, if not released frequently it can result in overdistension of the bladder, which increases the risk of infection. It also requires manual dexterity of patients (Fader et al. 1997). At night the catheter valve can be attached to an overnight bag, which allows the patient to get a good night's sleep (German et al. 1997).

Catheterization

Catheterization of males and females, although an invasive proce-dure, is a relatively simple one, providing it is performed by appro-priately trained personnel, which includes nurses, medical practitioners, carers and even the patient's partner (Willis 1995a). Introduction of the catheter by an unskilled practitioner can result in unnecessary trauma and possibly even strictures (Lowthian 1998; Woodward 1997).

There has been much controversy over the catheterization of males by female nurses and only in the 1990s has the restriction on this practice been lifted. Unless the patient requests otherwise, there is no reason to prevent a female nurse from catheterizing a male patient, provided the nurse has had the appropriate training and assessment, and is working within the UKCC Scope of Professional Practice in accordance with local health authority policies (RCN 1997; UKCC 1992; Winder 1994).

Consequently, the RCN (1997) has set out a number of guidelines pertaining to male catheterization:

1 The practitioner must have patient's permission or consent.
2 The practitioner must seek medical advice if there is a history of

recent surgery, trauma to the pelvis or abdomen, or congenital abnormalities.

3 The practitioner must be aware of product liability (expiry date and manufacturer's instructions).

4 There must be continuing care following catheterization.

There follows a breakdown of each step of the catheterization process, with a discussion or rationale as necessary, starting with female catheterization.

Female catheterization

Equipment

- lamp or adequate lighting
- plastic apron
- catheter pack
- sterile gloves (2 pairs)
- lignocaine gel or anaesthetic gel
- choice of catheter and spare
- syringe and needle
- sterile water
- catheter stand
- drainage bag.

Procedure

1. Gain the patient's permission/consent; ensure that the perineum is socially clean.
2. Explain the procedure and ensure lighting is adequate. (To reduce anxiety and facilitate cooperation.)
3. Use the treatment room if possible, if not then screen the bed. (To provide privacy and preserve the patient's dignity.)
4. Using aseptic technique, prepare the trolley and put on an apron.
5. Position the patient with her hips and knees flexed and apart. Maintain the patient's comfort.
6. Wash and dry your hands, and follow this with use of an antiseptic handrub. Allow assistant to open the packages on to the sterile trolley. The practitioner, wearing sterile gloves, prepares the sterile field. (To reduce cross infection; Lowthian 1998.)

7. With one hand, and using sterile gauze swabs, separate the labia. With the other hand, using separate sterile cotton wool for each stroke, clean the outer and inner aspects of the labia majora and labia minora. This must always be done in one direction going away from the urethra from front to back, with the final stroke down the urethral orifice. The use of antiseptics should be avoided (Lowthian 1998).

8. Change sterile gloves and position sterile towels.

9. Ensure that the correct volume of sterile water is drawn up in the syringe for balloon inflation according to the manufacturer's instructions.

10. Use the inner wrapping of the catheter as a collecting bag for urine, by partly sliding the bag down the catheter to expose the catheter tip.

11. Lubricate the catheter tip with sterile, single use, anaesthetic gel. (Anaesthetic gels are contraindicated in frequent catheterization, e.g. clean intermittent catheterization, due to the possibility of overdosing. The use of anaesthetic gels is often omitted in female catheterization. MacKenzie and Webb (1995) suggest that this is more to do with convention rather than research-based practice.)

12. Separate the labia using sterile gauze swabs and, using a clean gloved hand, insert the catheter into the urethral orifice. Maintain sterility of the catheter during insertion by slowly withdrawing it from the protective packaging only as it is inserted into the urethra (Willis 1998). The correct position will be indicated by the flow of urine into the catheter sleeve. If no urine flows check the catheter position, and if it is in the vagina then leave it in place until the second catheter has successfully been passed.

13. Instil the correct amount of water into the balloon channel.

14. Attach the catheter to the drainage system and support it on the stand or attach it to the patient's thigh.

15. Measure and record the residual volume of urine in the bladder.

16. Make the patient comfortable, providing explanations as required.

17. Dispose of all equipment correctly and wash your hands.

18. Document in the nursing records the type and size of catheter used.

Male catheterization (Figure 11.8)

Equipment

- lamp or adequate lighting
- plastic apron
- catheter pack
- sterile gloves (2 pairs)
- lignocaine gel or anaesthetic gel
- choice of catheter and spare
- syringe and needle
- sterile water
- catheter stand
- drainage bag.

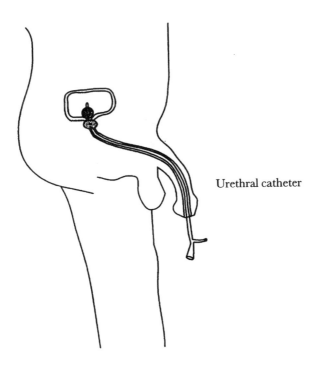

Urethral catheter

Figure 11.8 Male catheter (urethral).

Procedure

1.   Gain the patient's permission/consent; ensure that the meatus is socially clean.
2.   Explain the procedure and ensure lighting is adequate. (To reduce anxiety and facilitate cooperation.)
3.   Use the treatment room if possible, if not then screen the bed. (To provide privacy and preserve the patient's dignity.)
4.   Using aseptic technique, prepare the trolley and put on an apron.
5.   Maintain the patient's comfort.
6.   Wash and dry your hands, and follow this with use of an antiseptic handrub. Allow assistant to open the packages on to the sterile trolley. The practitioner, wearing sterile gloves, prepares the sterile field. (To reduce cross infection; Lowthian 1998.)
7.   Hold the penis with sterile gauze swabs, retracting the prepuce slightly to expose the urethral opening in non-circumcized patients. With the other hand clean the glans penis thoroughly using forceps and cotton wool.
8.   Change sterile gloves and position sterile towels.
9.   Ensure that the correct volume of sterile water is drawn up in the syringe for balloon inflation according to the manufacturer's instructions.
10. Use the inner wrapping of the catheter as a collecting bag for urine, by partly sliding the bag down the catheter to expose the catheter tip.
11. Instil lignocaine gel into the urethra, hold glans penis firmly to prevent the gel from being released and wait 2–3 minutes for the gel to take effect.
12. Using gauze, hold the penis in one hand, while introducing the catheter into the urethral meatus with the other hand. Guide the catheter slowly but smoothly until it passes into the bladder; this will be evident by a flow of urine. If resistance is felt at the prostate or sphincter region, elevate the penis to a 90 degree angle to the body and rotate the catheter slightly while inserting. Alternatively, asking the patient to relax his muscles as if passing urine, or to cough, will have the same effect. The catheter should never be forced.
13. Once urine is flowing, pass the catheter a further 5 cm to ensure the balloon is in the bladder. Never inflate the balloon

until urine is free-flowing. (All suprapubic and urethral catheterization should be performed when urine is present in the bladder. This reduces the chances of going into the ureter or unknowingly inflating the balloon in the urethra; Lowthian 1998.)

14. Inflate the balloon with the specific amount of water, asking the patient to report any pain felt while inflating the balloon (RCN 1997).
15. Replace prepuce if retracted to prevent paraphimosis (RCN 1997).
16. Attach the catheter to the drainage system and support it on the stand or attach it to the patient's thigh.
17. Measure and record the residual volume of urine in the bladder.
18. Make the patient comfortable, providing explanations as required.
19. Dispose of all equipment correctly and wash your hands.
20. Document in the nursing records the type and size of catheter used.

Suprapubic catheterization

As discussed above, initial suprapubic catheterization will almost certainly be performed by a doctor (Figure 11.9). However, the change of a suprapubic catheter can, according to local health authority policy, fall into the remit of the nurse. The RCN (1997) has provided guidelines for first-time catheter changes, as follows:

1. Adhere to full aseptic techniques.
2. Ensure that the bladder is easily palpable.
3. Following removal of the old catheter, a new catheter should be inserted immediately to prevent the closure of the original track.
4. As the new catheter is introduced resistance will ease as the catheter enters the bladder.
5. Insert the catheter further than the previous one and then half-fill the balloon. Gently withdraw until firm against the bladder wall and then completely inflate.
6. Occasionally urine does not drain immediately. Movement or coughing can initiate drainage.
7. Connect to the chosen drainage system.
8. Apply small dressing if required.
   (RCN 1997).

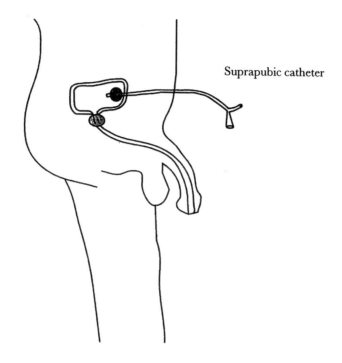

Figure 11.9 Male catheter (suprapubic).

Clean intermittent catheterization

All patients require a thorough assessment and discussion of needs and a clear explanation of the technique before starting intermittent catheterization (Cowan 1997; Winn and Thompson 1998). They should be given the opportunity to read supporting literature and watch video recordings of the technique, and be allowed to handle the catheter (RCN 1997). Prior to catheterization a patient should have established a suitable environment, the appropriate positioning and frequency of catheterization, and he or she should also be encouraged to void before catheterization (RCN 1997).

Clean intermittent catheterization is performed as urethral catheterization but as the name suggests, when it is performed by the patient or carer in the patient's own home the technique does not have to be aseptic, just clean. Within the hospital environment the technique should be carried out aseptically. There is no balloon to be inflated, instead the catheter is held in place until the urine flow stops and the bladder empties. The catheter is then withdrawn slowly.

Some intermittent catheters are coated with a special coating so that immersion into water causes the catheter to become slippery thus negating the need for anaesthetic lubricating gels. These catheters are disposable. However, some are designed to be used repeatedly and thus must be washed and dried thoroughly before being placed into storage.

Catheter management

Catheterization is an ongoing process, requiring long-term management in which nurses have a vital role. The aims of catheter management are:

- to promote patient dignity and comfort
- to minimize risk of secondary complications, e.g. tissue damage, infection, encrustation or blockage
- to help the patient to achieve a level of independence and self-care suitable for him or her
- to provide a cost-effective service (Getliffe 1996a; Winn 1996).

Psychological issues

The subject of continence is a highly sensitive and personal one. Nurses do not always deal with it appropriately, frequently addressing the topic in busy hospital wards in the presence of other patients and visitors (Roper et al. 1990). Long-term catheterization can allow many patients to gain control of their urinary dysfunction and re-engage in social activities without the fear of embarrassment. For other individuals it represents the difference between remaining in their own home and entering a residential or nursing home (Getliffe 1996a). Alternatively, a long-term catheter can impact and interfere with everyday living (Wilde 1997; Winn 1996). Wherever possible, patients and carers should be encouraged to enter into a partnership with the healthcare professional and be involved from the decision to catheterize, through to the long-term management (Willis 1995a; Woollons 1996).

Peate (1997) highlighted some patients' concerns regarding suprapubic catheterization. They are also pertinent to urethral catheters, as supported by Wilde (1997):

- loss of normal body function
- potential smells or odours

- leakage
- visibility of drainage bag and ability to empty bag when out
- sexual activity.

A study by German et al. (1997) supports some of the anxieties expressed by patients regarding drainage bags, including urine 'sloshing about' and the cumbersome, heavy bag which moves down the leg as it fills.

Sexual activity is an area often ignored by healthcare professionals, but patients should be aware that sexual activity need not stop. Urethral catheters should not be seen as a precluder to sexual activity, although with highly sexually active males other methods of catheterization, such as suprapubic or intermittent, should be considered, as there is the possibility of urethral trauma, possibly leading to stricture (Winder 1994). Men should be advised to fold the catheter back along the penis so that a condom can be worn over the top, and women should be shown how to reposition and tape the drainage bag to their abdomen (Getliffe 1996a; Rigby 1998). Alternatively, the patient can be taught how to remove and replace the old catheter with a new one following sexual activity (Winder 1994; Winson 1997).

Education has a significant effect on patients' acceptance of catheters (Winn 1996). This programme should begin prior to catheterization and should include how the catheter is positioned in the bladder and what it looks like with the balloon inflated. This should be supported by the use of booklets and videos, which are often supplied by the catheter manufacturers (Rigby 1998). However, sympathetic and skilful nursing is also essential in helping patients come to terms with long-term catheterization (Roper et al. 1990). Management should be seen as ongoing, with recognition that a patient's needs will change over time (Laurent 1998). Therefore nurses must undertake the dual roles of teacher and health educator, to offer support and provide adequate information to patients and carers whenever necessary (Roper et al. 1990).

Concluding remarks

Readers are encouraged to access the wealth of literature available on catheterization. The literature suggests that nurses frequently fail to base their clinical decisions on research evidence, action which is imperative when considering catheter type and selection since it is the nurse who is increasingly responsible for selecting catheters for patients.

The decision to catheterize must not be made to save on the nursing time of incontinent patients and must always be in their best interests. Catheterization carries with it a number of associated risks, but with the correct catheter choice following a full patient assessment, ongoing management and evaluation, these risks can be minimized.

For many patients a catheter is the difference between residential or nursing care and remaining in their own home, and consequently nurses must ensure that the catheter relieves their problems and does not exacerbate them.

Chapter 12
Patient education and nursing documentation

ANDREA GRIFFIN

Introduction

The new philosophy for healthcare aims to foster independence and promote health and autonomy among patients. Thus patient-centred care is rapidly evolving from ideology to reality. Patients are no longer considered as passive recipients of care and are encouraged to be actively involved in their own healthcare. Patient care is becoming holistic and individualized, and self-determination and patient choice are priorities.

For nurses this has meant a redesign and interpretation of their role. Traditional nurturing qualities of nursing that are thought to promote dependence among patients are no longer relevant. Task orientation and routinized care are inappropriate in the age of patient-centred care. Thus a number of practicable strategies, such as primary nursing and patient advocacy, have been developed in an attempt to achieve the goal of patient-centred care (Porter 1994). In addition, the relationship between nurse and patient has been replaced by a more egalitarian form of interaction, which promotes active participation of patients in their care (Porter 1994). This is known as the nurse–patient partnership. This style of nursing is thought to provide high-quality patient care and to make nursing a more satisfying experience for nurses themselves (May 1995).

The new healthcare and nursing philosophies are applicable to nursing in any urological setting. Urology is a dynamic and eclectic field of medicine, which incorporates a multitude of medical, surgical and oncological patients. It is therefore appropriate that nurses working in urology are aware of the philosophy in healthcare and are able to devise and execute strategies that achieve patient-centred care and fulfil the nurse–patient partnership. Therefore, outlining how the care of the urology patient can be improved and, equally, how the work experience of the urology nurse can be fulfilling, are important issues for discussion. This chapter will focus on patient empowerment, patient education and nursing documentation as a means to achieving the nurse–patient partnership and patient-centred care.

Empowering the patient

Patient empowerment has achieved popular status in recent nursing literature. It is part of the new dimension in nursing, which aims to achieve an equal partnership between nurse and patient. Rodwell (1996) defines empowerment as 'a helping process; a partnership valuing self and others; mutual decision-making and a freedom to make choices and accept responsibility'. Similarly, empowerment is described as a 'process of helping people to assert control over the factors which affect their lives' (Gibson 1991). Empowerment is seen as a process that involves the sharing of resources (Gibson 1991) and the transfer of power (Rodwell 1996). Empowerment is about giving patients the means to take responsibility for their own health. It is therefore essential that in order to empower patients, nurses must be empowered themselves (Rodwell 1996; Chavesse 1992).

Information and empowerment

Information is central to the empowerment process. Research has shown that information is an essential need among cancer patients (Ream and Richardson 1996) and that, similarly, most patients with cancer wish to receive information about their illness, whether this be good or bad (Hinds et al. 1995). With information, patients are suitably equipped to make a choice, to be involved in decision making and to accept responsibility for their healthcare needs. Thus much research has focused on the information preferences of patients. In studies concerning cancer patients, information has been identified as a major source of personal control for patients to cope with their illness (Davison and Degner 1997). Information has been shown to have other benefits for cancer patients, such as increasing participation in decision making (Cassileth et al. 1980; Hinds et al. 1995; Davison and Degner 1997), reducing stress and anxiety (Cassileth et al. 1980; Hinds et al. 1995; Ream and Richardson 1996), increasing treatment compliance (Hinds et al. 1995) and increasing hope (Cassileth et al. 1980).

Empowerment and choice

Although many patients have expressed a need for information, in reality not all patients desire detailed information about their illness and its treatment and they may refuse responsibility and participation in decision making altogether. Similarly, those patients who want to be informed may not receive the information they want or they may receive an excess of information that they cannot retain (Jakobsson et al. 1997). In these situations, the empowerment process may be hindered or prove impossible. How can a patient who desires a passive role in his or her care possibly be empowered? Patient empowerment is an attractive concept but its implementation in a clinical setting may be problematic. However, perhaps the key element in the empowerment process is choice. When patients are given the freedom to choose whether or not they want information; whether they want to be an active or passive receiver of care, it can be argued that they have been empowered because they have been given a choice. Allowing patients the right to choose and respecting their decision upholds their autonomy and ultimately empowers the patient.

Empowering the urology patient

A study by Davison and Degner (1997) focused on men with prostate cancer and hypothesized that information would help the men obtain a more active role in decision making and reduce their stress and anxiety. The study showed how the men with newly diagnosed prostate cancer desired information, but were happy to designate decisional responsibility to their doctor. Six weeks on in the study, after having received an information package, the majority of the men wanted to be involved in their treatment decisions and 25% of these men wanted to select their own medical treatment. Davison and Degner (1997) suggest that the men's desire to be actively involved in their treatment stems from the information they received about their cancer and support from their families. Significantly, those men who chose to be involved in decision making had lower levels of anxiety than those who preferred a more passive role.

A study in Sweden by Jakobsson et al. (1997) focused on men with prostate cancer who were either active or passive receivers of care. Similarly, the passive receivers of care had difficulty expressing their needs to the nurses and appeared to suffer in silence. The active receivers of care were able to make contact with the nurses and discuss with them exactly what they needed. These patients felt that the nursing care they received met their needs.

Interpretation of the results of these studies would suggest that active receivers of care require sufficient information to enable them to become active and influential in their treatment and care. Being an active participant has positive outcomes, such as reduced anxiety levels and the ability to express needs adequately. Passive receivers of care may have increased anxiety levels and an inability to express their needs. Another issue arising from the study by Davison and Degner (1997) is that active participation is not necessarily a static concept, since patients changed from being passive to active receivers of care. This suggests that patients should always be offered a choice about the information they want to receive and the type of involvement they desire. Health professionals should be aware that patients may be liable to change their minds about their care at any stage of their treatment. It is therefore appropriate that information and the freedom to choose are a realistic option for all patients throughout their illness career.

Empowering the urology patient then, is a process that must include choice for patients. Information must be given to patients who desire it, at an appropriate and manageable level. Patients should be allowed to participate in treatment decisions and in their care if they so wish. If a patient prefers a passive role, his or her wish should be respected, but they should not be neglected and should be informed of any alternatives and the benefits they may bring.

Autonomy and informed consent

Autonomy is closely related to empowerment and choice. Where empowerment is concerned with offering patients choice, autonomy is about respecting the choices made by patients. Autonomy arises from the utilitarian and deontological ethical theories, which claim that there is a moral requirement to respect a person's autonomy

(Willard 1995). Consequently, respecting a patient's autonomy has achieved recognition as an essential component of effective nursing care.

Informed consent is a tangible expression of autonomy. Informed consent has been defined as 'a voluntary, uncoerced decision, made by a sufficiently competent or autonomous person on the basis of adequate information and deliberation, to accept rather than reject some proposed course of action that will affect him or her' (Gillon 1985). Informed consent is a process of shared decision making, based on mutual respect and participation, involving more than the ritual reading of a form (Molin 1996). The UKCC states that one must obtain consent before giving any treatment or care. In some cases consent can obtained verbally, but for invasive or surgical procedures, written consent is required. True informed consent can only be achieved when adequate information is given to the patient, so that they can accept or refuse treatment based on their knowledge of it.

However, defining exactly what constitutes 'adequate information' is problematic. Two opposing perspectives have arisen over the disclosure of information for informed consent. One perspective adopts a paternalistic stance, believing that patients are unnecessarily distressed by too much information (Willard 1995). The second perspective actively encourages the disclosure of information to patients, because it not only supports patient autonomy, but also helps to reduce patient anxiety (Teasdale 1993).

Research by Kerrigan et al. (1993) addressed the notion that patients would become unduly anxious if given detailed information about the risks of surgery during informed consent. The results showed that detailed information, including an explanation about undergoing surgery, did not increase patient anxiety. Kerrigan et al. (1993) concluded that giving detailed information prior to obtaining informed consent has the advantage of allowing patients fully informed consent before they consent to surgery, thus reducing the potential for subsequent litigation. However, research by Lavelle-Jones et al. (1993) examined the factors influencing the quality of informed consent and found that patients had difficulty recalling the information after signing their consent form. Sixty-nine percent of the study also admitted to not reading the consent form before signing. Lavelle-Jones et al. (1993) concluded that in order to improve patients' recall of information, written information should be given to patients prior to admission to hospital.

Interpretation of the current research in informed consent suggests that patients, including urology patients, may benefit from receiving detailed information about treatments, since this empowers them to make an informed choice. Information should be provided both verbally and in written form to maximize patient recall of information.

Patient education

Information has been identified as an essential need for patients. Thus, patient education has featured considerably in nursing literature over the past 25 years (Redman 1993). Patient education has been defined as 'a process assisting people to learn and incorporate health-related behaviours into everyday life' (Smith 1989). The intention of patient education is to bring about behavioural and attitudinal changes in patients (Luker and Caress 1989). Successful patient education assists patients to become partners in their medical care regimens and fit new health behaviours into their daily activities (Smith 1989). Although patient education and patient teaching are often used interchangeably, a distinction can be drawn between the two. Rankin and Duffy (1983) describe patient teaching as a component of patient education that refers to the imparting of information only.

Although patient education has received popular status in nursing literature, there is much debate concerning the extent to which patient education is indeed a nursing responsibility. Similarly the most appropriate and effective medium through which to deliver information is also unclear. It is therefore appropriate that these issues are discussed further, since patient education may be crucial in the empowerment of patients and in fulfilling the nurse–patient partnership. It is also significant to explore patient education and its relationship in a urological setting, since many urological procedures, such as clean intermittent self-catheterization (CISC), require education from a health professional.

Current trends in healthcare, which favour health promotion and autonomy among patients, have increased the need for patient education. Patients are encouraged to take responsibility for their own healthcare needs and to do this they require informational input from a health professional. In addition, there is evidence to suggest that patient education improves compliance with treatment and consequently health and well being (Cohen 1981). Patient education appears to have both physical and psychological benefits for patients (Luker and Caress 1989) and is thus a desirable component of patient care.

Ideally patient education should involve planning and be a well structured event. Close (1987) suggests that the teaching process can be compared to the nursing process, i.e. involving assessment, planning, implementation and evaluation. Assessment will enable the nurse to discover exactly what the patient wants and needs to know, thus ensuring individuality (Wilson-Barnett 1985). An assessment of the patient will also enable the nurse to determine the patient's readiness to learn, since the attitude and the motivation of the patient may be a barrier to successful learning. Close (1987) suggests that assessment will provide the opportunity for goal setting between the nurse and patient. The goals should state a realistic aim of what the patient should be able to achieve at the end of the teaching sessions.

Adult education

The structure of patient education as described by Close (1987), reflects the principles of andragogy. 'Andragogy' is the art and science of helping adults to learn (Knowles 1980). The principles of andragogy stem from the belief that adult education and initial education are fundamentally different processes. Knowles (1980) explains this by the change in personality as a person matures, where there is a move from a dependent personality towards one of a self-directing human being. A learning environment where the teacher transmits knowledge to the learner; where learning is a one-way process, is not conducive to adult learning. An adult needs to be self-directing, with formal teaching replaced by mutual inquiry and the learner in control of what is to be learnt and how this will be achieved. Knowles (1980) suggests that the learner should be involved in planning his or her own learning and formulating his or her own learning objectives.

Knowles (1980) explains that an adult accumulates a growing reservoir of experience, which is a rich resource for learning. It is believed that adults like to learn from experience, since personal experiences establish self-identity and so are highly valued (Knowles 1980). Thus emphasis should be directed towards a practical approach to learning, such as group discussion, simulation exercises and problem-solving activities (Knowles 1980).

The role of the teacher in adult education is that of a facilitator. As a facilitator, learning becomes a process of mutual inquiry, where the facilitator's aim is to assist the learners to become self-directed (Neilson 1992). It is expected that the facilitator should have expertise in the subject area and be able to offer guidance and support (D'A Slevin and Lavery 1991). As a facilitator, the nurse should aim to encourage the patient to take responsibility for his or her own learning, thereby reducing dependence on the nurse and ultimately preparing the patient for the transition from hospital to home.

The principles of adult education and andragogy have important implications for patient education. If adults prefer to be self-directed, practical learners, then adult patient education should reflect this. In addition, nurses as educators should adopt the facilitator approach to teaching. Indeed Close (1987) suggests that nurses should be familiar with the theories of teaching and learning. Patient education should, therefore, follow the direction of self-directed learning and aim to encourage patients to have control over what they learn, with the guidance and support of the facilitator.

The role of the nurse in patient education

Although a framework for successful patient education exists, the extent to which patient education and patient teaching are practised by nurses remains unclear (Redman 1993). A review of the literature by Close (1987) concluded that despite nurses recognizing patient teaching as part of their role, effective patient teaching was not taking place. A number of reasons may exist to explain this. Luker and Caress (1989) identify length of stay in hospital as a barrier to successful patient education, where planned patient education is upset when patients are discharged unexpectedly. Lack of time, heavy workload and inadequate staffing have also been cited as reasons, indeed Luker and Caress (1989) state that it is doubtful if teaching skills can be fully integrated as part of everyday nursing work.

The patients themselves may also prove to be a barrier to learning, since psychological changes that accompany illness may affect their capacity to learn. In an acute setting such as a urology ward, patients are in a difficult environment, at a time when they may be anxious or in pain. Such constraints on learning and teaching appear to highlight the difficulties faced by nurses when implementing patient education into patient care. Thus, expecting nurses to partake in patient education as part of their everyday role may be unrealistic and impossible to achieve.

Research on patient education in nursing has revealed that an incongruity exists between nurses and patients regarding their perceptions of the role of the nurse in patient education. A review of the literature by Close (1987) revealed that patients did not often identify the nurse as the most valuable source of information or somebody capable of teaching patients. Similar results were found in a study by Tilley et al. (1987), where patients stated that although they recognized a general teaching function for nurses, they preferred to be taught by a physician. Nurses identified themselves as the most desirable patient teacher and incorrectly assumed the type of information most valuable to patients. As a result of these findings Tilley et al. (1987) suggest that nurses need to develop a clear definition of their role in patient education.

The UKCC guidelines for professional practice stress the professional role of the nurse in promoting autonomy and independence of patients through the provision of adequate information. Although patient education is not formally mentioned here, the imparting of information implies that patient teaching is a necessary component of effective nursing care. Luker and Caress (1989) also recognize the nurse as a valuable source of information for patients, but question nurses' ability to assess whether information has been received and understood by the patient. They suggest that patient education may be more suited to the role of specialist nurses, who have both the interest and the specialist knowledge to make them ideal patient educators.

Perhaps then, in an acute setting such as a urology ward, where patient education may be an unrealistic goal for general nurses, specialist nurses could fulfil this responsibility. The specialist nurse may be able to devote more time to comprehensive procedures, such as CISC and stoma care. The general nurse, therefore, has an important role in patient teaching, such as discussing proposed treatment options, postoperative care and pain control. Nurses also have a responsibility to provide written information, which is known to be highly valued by patients (Griffiths and Leek 1995; Hinds et al. 1995).

New directions in patient education

New directions in patient education consider andragogical principles and have placed the responsibility of learning on to the patient. One example of a self-directed approach to patient education is computer-assisted learning (CAL). By using a learning package on a computer, patients are able to work through information at their own pace and complete problem-solving exercises in simulated situations. A review of research evaluating the effectiveness of CAL by Luker and Caress (1989) has revealed favourable results, with CAL described as a useful way of educating patients. Even those patients who may be unfamiliar with computers and a keyboard can benefit from CAL, since much of the software requires patients to use just one or two keys (Luker and Caress 1989). It is therefore also beneficial to patients with literacy problems (Luker and Caress 1989).

Self-directed approaches to patient education, such as computer-assisted learning, demonstrate how nurses can transfer the responsibility of learning to the patient. It is intended for self-directed approaches to reduce the patient's dependency upon the nurse, thereby promoting independence and autonomy among patients.

Nursing documentation

Documentation of the nursing care given to patients is a compulsory component of everyday nursing. Ensuring that nursing documentation is of a high standard is of increasing importance, since nurses are accountable for their actions. Good documentation should ensure a smooth transition between change over of nurses and a degree of continuity for patients.

Exactly how documentation can empower patients and achieve the nurse–patient partnership is not strikingly obvious. However, one method of documentation – the integrated care pathway – aims to benefit patients as well as all members of the multidisciplinary team. In our area of work an integrated care pathway for the transurethral resection of prostate (TURP) or bladder tumour (TURBT) has been developed and piloted. It is hoped that this form of documentation will improve the standard of care given to patients, improve communication between health professionals and reduce any unnecessary length of stay in hospital for patients. This section focuses on integrated care pathways and provides examples of how they can be used in a urological setting.

An integrated care pathway (Figure 12.1), which can also be referred to as a critical pathway or clinical pathway, is a pre-printed document that sets out the treatment and clinical goals for the patient on a daily basis. The care pathway is diagnosis- or procedure-based, such as a pathway for myocardial infarction or for a surgical procedure such as TURP. The overall aim of the document is to enable collaboration between members of the multidisciplinary team, where all team members work together towards a common goal (Wigfield and Boon 1996).

Patient Problem/Focus	Post-op day of surgery Date	First day post-op Date
Assessment	Goal: No problems following surgery. Vital signs within acceptable limits Monitored as necessary Goal: Bladder irrigation running status as per protocol Reduced Yes ☐ No ☐ In & Output measured & recorded regularly Colour of drainage/Degree of Haematuria acceptable ☐ Observe for abdominal distention/increase in pain to exclude clot retention Catheter secure ☐ Patient not c/o spasm ☐ Anti-cholinergic prescribed ☐ Analgesia adequate Yes ☐ No ☐ IVI maintained ☐ IVI discontinued ☐ Venflon left in situ until Hb result known ☐	Goal: No problems following surgery. Assessed by medical staff ☐ Vital signs within acceptable limits temp < 37° Bladder irrigation running status as per protocol Discontinued if colour of drainage/Degree of Haematuria acceptable @ .... ☐ In & Output measured & recorded regularly. Total for last 24 hrs ...... (@ 12mm) Catheter to be removed at 12 midnight Yes ☐ No ☐ No signs of distention, clots, TUR. Syndrome ☐ Analgesia adequate Yes ☐ No ☐ IVI discontinued ☐ Venflon left in situ until Hb result known ☐ Bowels open Yes ☐ No ☐ Aperient given Yes ☐ No☐ No evidence of DVT or PE
Individual patient problem		
Investigations		Check Hb, U & E
Treatments/ Procedures	Change gown & freshen up catheter care maintained 4 hrly	Goal: catheter removed at midnight Yes ☐ No ☐ catheter care maintained 4 hrly by patient ☐ Nurse ☐ Catheter secure ☐ Hygiene needs met TEDS removed and replaced

Continued

Mobility/ Safety	Goal: Risk/fall minimised post op Call bell is accessible to patient Encouraged to move legs & do deep breathing exercises when recovered from anaesthetic	Patient sits out of bed Encouraged to mobilise to usual ability
Medication	Pain is scored & analgesia given Nausea & vomiting treated if present Anti-cholingeric given as prescribed	Pain is scored and analgesia given Anti-cholingeric given as prescribed Aperient given if required
Patient Problem/Focus	Post-op day of surgery Date	First day post-op Date
Diet	Fluids and light diet tolerated Treat nausea/vomiting if present	Goal: Normal diet tolerated Fluids encouraged (2–3 litres per day)
Psychosocial/ Teaching	Reassurance given	Goal: Patient understands the operation performed Pt encouraged to ask questions and express any fears or anxieties information reinforced
Discharge Planning		
If you cannot sign off a goal please describe variance & state action on progress notes before signing below.		
Please sign each shift	Early .... Late .... Night	Early .... Late .... Night ....

Figure 12.1 Integrated pathway for transurethral resection of prostate

The pathway adopts a format of a Gnatt chart, which outlines the patient's suggested care process on a time-task matrix (Pearson et al. 1995). The day-to-day treatment and clinical goals are based on interdisciplinary standards and evidence-based practice. All members of the multidisciplinary team are requested to evaluate and document care on the pathway, which therefore replaces individual forms of documentation. It is intended that the document be placed at the patient's bedside and is thus available for the use of the patient and his or her family. The specific goals of care pathways usually include the following:

- Selecting a 'best practice', when practice styles vary unnecessarily.
- Defining standards for the expected duration of hospital stay and for the use of tests and treatments.
- Examining the interrelations among the different steps in the care

process to find ways to coordinate or to decrease time spent in the rate-limiting steps.

- Giving all hospital staff a common 'game plan' from which to view and understand their various roles in the overall care process.
- Providing a framework for collecting data on the care process so that providers can learn how often and why patients do not follow an expected course during their hospitalization.
- Decreasing nursing and physician documentation burdens.
- Improving patient satisfaction with care by educating patients and their families about the plan of care and involving them more fully in its implementation (Pearson et al. 1995).

An important feature of the care pathway is the documentation of any variance from care. A variance refers to anything that occurs which is not planned or anticipated on the pathway (Hotchkiss 1997). Individualized patient care means that variances are to be expected and do not, therefore, necessarily mean bad practice (Wigfield and Boon 1996). The documentation of all variance provides a wealth of information for data analysis and it is this analysis of variance on which future changes and improvements in care will be based. Variance analysis, therefore, places critical pathways squarely within the tradition of continuous quality improvement (Pearson et al. 1995).

Although integrated care pathways have achieved favourable reviews in recent nursing and medical literature, certain concerns about autonomy, individualized care, litigation and effectiveness have arisen. Since care pathways are standardized, dictating patient care and patient goals, it is argued that the patient's autonomy is threatened. Pearson et al. (1995) argue that physicians may gain greater control over their patients by helping to define those standards included on the pathway. Patient involvement in the pathway may help to increase their autonomy. Patients should be invited to read the pathway and use it as a source of information, providing a plan of what to expect during their stay in hospital.

Similarly, it has been suggested that since pathways are pre-printed and diagnosis-led, they do not constitute individualized care (Hotchkiss 1997). However, the fact that the pathway accounts for, and actively encourages the documentation of, variance suggests that patients do not have to strictly adhere to the pathway. The pathway is a flexible document because it anticipates that the care of each patient will be different. Analysis of variance data will contribute to future pathways, ensuring that patient care will continue to be as individualized as possible.

Another concern raised about care pathways is that health professionals may feel more vulnerable to malpractice suits if they do not comply with the care stated on the care pathway and a complication occurs (Pearson et al. 1995). However, in practice an increase in litigation has not been reported from centres in the USA or in Britain using multidisciplinary care planning (Hotchkiss 1997). In fact, care pathways may increase the case for the defence for several reasons. First, the pathway sets out a clear plan of the treatment and goals to be achieved. Completion of the pathway will provide evidence of whether or not the plan was followed and, if not, what alternative action was taken (Hotchkiss 1997). In addition, a common complaint received from patients is the lack of communication that occurs during their stay in hospital (Hotchkiss 1997). The care pathway attempts to improve communication between multidisciplinary members and also between patients and health professionals, thereby recognizing the importance of communication between patients and staff.

Despite the implementation of care pathways in clinical practice, uncertainty persists regarding their effectiveness (Pearson et al. 1997). Pearson et al. (1997), state that the research which suggests that care pathways decrease hospital stay for patients is sparse and that there is little research data available about the costs, implementation and maintenance of care pathways.

One problem encountered by Wigfield and Boon (1996) was that users forgot or stated that they were too busy to complete the pathway. Similarly, it was found that some members of the multidisciplinary team were reluctant to complete the pathway and preferred to document in the traditional style of the case notes. Wigfield and Boon (1996) emphasize the importance of having a coordinator or link person for maintaining and motivating the project. This should ensure smooth implementation of the pathway, where all members of the multidisciplinary team are confident in using and completing the pathway. The potential benefits of care pathways have been summarized as follows:

- More information is available for patients and clinicians.
- There is a reduction in documentation and in duplication of documentation.

- They aid in the facilitation of staff education/induction programmes.
- The appropriate average length of stay can be determined through the reduction in variance (Hothchkiss 1997).

Using care pathways in a urological setting

In the USA, a series of studies has been conducted focusing on care pathways in a variety of urological operations, including more complex operations such as radical retropubic prostatectomy, cystectomy and cystoprostatectomy. The overall aim of the development of these pathways was to investigate if collaborative care methods could affect hospital costs, duration of stay in hospital for patients and improve the quality of care given to patients.

Koch et al. (1995) introduced a collaborative care pathway for cystectomy and urinary reconstruction. The care pathway was used as a means of standardizing care and minimizing insufficient medical practices. This was achieved by eliminating those medical practices that had become established through precedent and lacked justification in the literature (Koch et al. 1995). A clinical nurse specialist was involved in identifying and documenting the current norms for clinical course and management for cystectomy and urinary reconstruction. The development of an integrated care pathway for this procedure was seen as a challenge for the authors, since it is a complex operation with relatively high morbidity and mortality rates. The results of the study were compared with the results for patients who had undergone radical cystectomy prior to the implementation of the pathway.

The results of the study showed that hospital charges decreased and the duration in hospital for patients decreased from 12.7 days to 10.3 days. There were also decreases in the duration of surgery, blood loss, intensive care unit use and postoperative morbidity rates. Koch et al. (1995) concluded that collaborative care pathways favourably affect the cost efficiency of care and provide favourable surgical outcomes. Any initial concerns that the radical cystectomy patient population and procedure were too complex to be managed with a collaborative care technique were unfounded. Therefore, Koch et al. (1995) state that collaborative care pathways are applicable to virtually all urological operations, with enormous potential to effect improvements in the quality and cost-efficiency of care.

A second study by Koch and Smith (1996) sought to establish if a collaborative care pathway was applicable to patients of different ages and co-morbidity. Patients older than 70 years and those with pathology such as hypertension, diabetes, myocardial infarction, COPD and cerebrovascular accident (CVA) were included in the study alongside patients younger than 70 with no other significant pathology. These patients underwent either radical prostatectomy or cystoprostatectomy, using a collaborative care approach and were compared to historical findings prior to the implementation of the pathway. Koch and Smith (1996) found that the standardized approach to patient care yielded excellent outcomes, despite the disparities between patients. This suggests that the pathway was sufficiently flexible to accommodate older and more ill patients, as well as younger, healthier patients (Koch and Smith 1996). This study shows that all patients are candidates for care pathways regardless of any past or existing medical history. Care pathways, therefore, have sufficient scope to accommodate a variety of patients and still produce successful results.

The results of the studies by Koch et al. (1995) and Koch and Smith (1996) should be interpreted with caution since relatively small numbers were involved in the sample and the results were compared to retrospective cases and thus a control group was not used. However, the studies clearly show that it is possible to construct a care pathway for a multitude of urological procedures and thus integrated care pathways have a place in urology and its future.

References

Ashford L (1998) Erectile dysfunction. Professional Nurse 13(9): 603–8.

Atwell JD (1997) Epidemiology and genetics of genitourinary malformations. In Thomas DFM (ed) Urological Disease in the Fetus and Infant Diagnosis and Management. Oxford: Butterworth-Heinemann.

Atzpodien J, Korfer A, Franks CR et al. (1990) Home therapy with recombinant inter-leukin-2 and interferon-alpha 2b in advanced human malignancies. Lancet 335: 1509–12.

Bakke A, Digranes A, Hoistaeter P (1997) Physical predictors of infection in patients treated with clean intermittent catheters: a prospective 7 year study. British Journal of Urology 79: 85–90.

Barnes K, Malone-Lee J (1986) Long-term catheter management: minimising problem of premature replacement due to balloon deflation. Journal of Advanced Nursing 11: 303–7.

Benjamin H (1966) The Transsexual Phenomenon. New York: The Julian Press.

Benjamin H (1981) Standards of Care: The Hormonal and Surgical Reassignment of Gender Dysphoric Persons. California: The Harry Benjamin International Gender Dysphoria Association Inc.

Blandy J (1991) Lecture Notes on Urology, 4th edn. London: Blackwell.

Bloom D, McGuire J, Lapides J (1994) A brief history of urethral catheterisation. The Journal of Urology 151: 317–25.

Brewster SF, Kemple T, MacIver AG et al. (1994) The Bristol prostate cancer pilot screening study: a three year follow up. British Journal of Urology 74: 556–8.

Britton E, Wright E (1996) Catheters: making an informed choice. Professional Nurse January: 194–8.

Bull E, Chilton CP, Gould AL, Sutton TM (1991) Single-blind, randomised, parallel group study of Bard Biocath catheter and a silicone elastomer coated catheter. British Journal of Urology 68: 394–9.

Bullock N, Sibley G, Whitaker R (1994) Essential Urology. London: Churchill Livingstone.

Burgers JK, Badalament RA et al. (1992) Penile cancer: clinical presentation, diagnosis and staging. Urologic Clinics of North America 19(2).

Burns D (1992) Working up a thirst. Nursing Times 88(26): 44–5.

Cancer Research Campaign (1991) Testicular Cancer – UK. Factsheet 16. London:

190

Cancer Research Campaign.

Carey P, Charlton A, Sloper P, White D (1995) Cancer education in secondary schools. Educational Review 47(1): 101–11.

Carney S, Karlowicz KA, Meredith C et al. (1995) Urinary tract symptoms. In Karlowicz KA (ed) Urologic Nursing: Principles and Practice. London: WB Saunders.

Cassileth BR, Zupkis DV, Sutton-Smith K, March V (1980) Information preferences among cancer patients. Annals of Internal Medicine 92: 832–6.

Chavesse J (1992) New dimensions of empowerment in nursing – and challenges. Journal of Advanced Nursing 17: 1–2.

Close A (1987) Patient education: a literature review. Journal of Advanced Nursing 13: 203–13.

Cockett ATK, Khoury S, Aso Y et al. (eds) (1993) Recommendations of the international consensus committee. In Proceedings of the Second International Consultation on Benign Prostatic Hyperplasia, Paris, 27–30 June.

Cohen SA (1981) Patient education – a review of the literature. Journal of Advanced Nursing 6: 11–18.

Cowan T (1997) Catheters designed for intermittent use. Professional Nurse 12(4): 297–302.

Cox AJ (1990) Comparison of catheter surface morphologies. British Journal of Urology 65: 55–60.

Crawford ED, Dawkins CA (1988) Cancer of the penis. In Skinner DG, Lieskovsky G (eds) Diagnosis and Management of Genitourinary Cancer. Philadelphia, PA: WB Saunders.

Crow R, Mulhall A, Chapman R (1998) Indwelling catheterisation and related nursing practice. Journal of Advanced Nursing 13: 489–95.

Cudow PM, Thomas DFM (1997) Duplication and other anomalies in the kidney and ureter. In Thomas DFM (ed) Urological Disease in the Fetus and Infant Diagnosis and Management. Oxford: Butterworth-Heinemann.

Cullinane C (1997) Pathology of the kidney and urinary tract in infancy. In Thomas DFM (ed) Urological Disease in the Fetus and Infant Diagnosis and Management. Oxford: Butterworth-Heinemann.

D'A Slevin O, Lavery M (1991) Self-directed learning and student supervision. Nurse Education Today 11: 368–77.

Davison J, Degner L (1997) Empowerment of men newly diagnosed with prostate cancer. Cancer Nursing 20(3): 187–96.

Dawson C, Whitfield H (1996) Common paediatric problems. British Medical Journal 312(7041): 1291–4.

Dawson C, Whitfield H (1997) ABC of Urology. London: British Medical Journal.

Denning J (1996) Transsexuality in the Workplace: A Guide For Managers Dealing With an Employee's Change of Gender Role. London: The Gender Trust.

Department of Health (1995) Hospital Episode Statistics 1994–95. London: HMSO.

Diabetes Control and Complications Group (1993) The effect of intensive treatment of diabetes on the development and progression of long term complications in insulin dependent diabetes mellitus. New England Journal of Medicine 329: 977–86.

Downey P, Dean M, Hayes J (1997) Perfect timing. Nursing Times 93(5): 89–90.

Downey P, Fordham M (1998) Bowel preparation in the pre op ileal conduit patient. The Royal Liverpool University Hospitals (unpublished).

Drummond MF, McGuire AJ, Black NA et al. (1993) Economic burden of treating benign prostatic hyperplasia in the United Kingdom. British Journal of Urology 71: 290–6.

Editorial (1995) Drugs and Therapy Perspectives 6: 5–7.

Fenwick E (1997) Urological cancers. In Fillingham S, Douglas J (eds) Urological Nursing, 2nd edn. London: Baillière Tindall.

Fillingham S, Douglas J (eds) (1997) Urological Nursing, 2nd edn. London: Baillière Tindall.

Fader M, Petterson L, Brooks R, Dean G, Wells M, Cottenden A, Malone-Lee J (1997) A multicentre comparative evaluation of catheter valves. British Journal of Nursing 6(7): 359–67.

Finlay T (1989) Fluid balance in patients undergoing major gut surgery. Surgical Nurse 4: 11–16.

Flannery M (1992) Reproductive Cancers: Core Curriculum for Oncology Nursing. Philadelphia, PA: WB Saunders.

Fonkalsrud EW (1996) Current management of the undescended testis. Seminars in Pediatric Surgery 5(1): 2–7.

Freedman ER, Rickwood AMK (1994) Urinary incontinence due to unilateral vaginal ectopic single ureters. British Journal of Urology 73: 716–17.

Garraway WM, Collins GN, Lee RJ (1991) High prevalence of benign prostatic hypertrophy in the community. Lancet 338: 469–71.

Garrett BM (1995) The nutritional management of acute renal failure. Journal of Clinical Nursing 4: 377–82.

Gauntlett-Beare P, Myers JL (1994) Adult Health Nursing, 2nd edn. St Louis: Mosby.

Gelder M, Goth D, Mayou R (1989) Oxford Text Book of Psychiatry, 2nd edn. Oxford University Press, p 591.

German K, Rowley P, Stone D, Kumar U, Blackford HN (1997) A randomised cross over study comparing the use of a catheter valve and a leg bag in urethrally catheterised male patients. British Journal of Urology 79: 96–8.

Getliffe K (1993) Informed choices for long-term benefits: the management of catheters in continence care. Professional Nurse 9(2): 122–6.

Getliffe K (1996) Care of urinary catheters. Nursing Standard 11(11): 47–50.

Gibbs T (1995) Health assessment of the adult urology patient. In Karlowicz KA (ed) Urologic Nursing: Principles and Practice. London: WB Saunders.

Gibson C (1991) A concept analysis of the concept of empowerment. Journal of Advanced Nursing 16: 354–61.

Gilbert HW, Gingell JC (1992) Vacuum constriction devices: second line conservative treatment for impotence. Journal of Urology 70: 81–3.

Gillon R (1985) Philosophical Medical Ethics. Chichester: Wiley and Sons.

Gingell JC (1998) Transurethral prostaglandin for erectile dysfunction. Trends in Urology, Gynaecology and Sexual Health May/Jun: 15–16.

Giroux JA (1995) Urinary tract infections in adults. In Karlowicz KA (ed) Urologic Nursing: Principles and Practice. London: WB Saunders.

Gleason DF, Mellinger GT (1974) Veterens administrations cooperative urological research group: prediction of prognosis for prostatic adenocarcinoma by histological grading and clinical staging. Journal of Urology 3: 58–64.

Grabstald H (1990) Controversies surrounding lymph node dissection for carcinoma penis. Urologic Clinics of North America 7.

Griffiths M, Leek C (1995) Patient education needs: opinions of oncology nurses and their patients. Oncology Nursing Forum 22(1): 139–43.

Hage JJ (1995) Metaidioplasty: an alternative phalloplasty technique in transsexuals. Plastic and Reconstructive Surgery 97(1): 161–7.

Hanno PM, Wein AJ (1994) Clinical Manual of Urology, 2nd edn. New York: McGraw Hill.

Harris DJ, Boyle MO, Warbrick C (1995) Law of the European Convention on Human Rights. London: Reed Elsevier, p 439.

Hinds C, Streater A, Mood D (1995) Funtions and preferred methods of receiving information related to radiotherapy. Cancer Nursing 18(5): 374–84.

Hodges C (1997) Continence care: choosing carefully. Nursing Times 93: 35.

Holmes SAV (1998a) Erectile dysfunction: part 1, epidemiology and causes. Trends in Urology, Gynaecology and Sexual Health Jan/Feb: 39–42

Holmes SAV (1998b) Erectile dysfunction: hospital management. Trends in Urology, Gynaecology and Sexual Health Jul/Aug: 20–4.

Hotchkiss R (1997) Integrated care pathways. Nursing Times Research 2(1): 30–6.

International Continence Society (1984) The Standardisation of Terminology of the Lower Urinary Tract Function. London: ICS.

Jakobsson L, Hallberg IR, Loven L (1997) Met and unmet nursing care needs in men with prostate cancer. An exploration study part 2. European Journal of Cancer Care 6: 117–23.

Johnson DE, Lo RK (1987) Tumours of the Penis, Urethra, and Scrotum: Genitourinary Cancer Management. Philadelphia, PA: Lea and Febiger.

Kennedy A, Brocklehurst J (1982) The nursing management of patients with long-term indwelling catheters. Journal of Advanced Nursing 7: 411–17.

Kerrigan D, Thevasgayam R, Woods T, McWelch I, Thomas W, Shorthouse A, Dennison A (1993) Who's afraid of informed consent? British Medical Journal 306: 298–300.

Kirby R (1997) Management of common prostatitis syndromes. Trends in Urology Gynaecology and Sexual Health Nov/Dec: 37–43.

Klimaszewski AD, Karlowicz KA (1995) In Karlowicz KA (ed) Urologic Nursing: Principles and Practice. London: WB Saunders.

Knowles MS (1980) The Modern Practice of Adult Education: From Pedagogy to Andragogy. Chicago: Association Press.

Koch M, Seckin B, Smith Jr J (1995) Impact of a collaborative care approach to radical cystectomy and urinary reconstruction. Journal of Urology 154: 996–1001.

Koch M, Smith Jr J (1996) Influence of patient age and co-morbidity on outcome of a collaborative care pathway after radical prostatectomy and cystoprostatectomy. Journal of Urology 155: 1681–4.

Kohler-Ockmore J (1991) Chronic urinary catheter blockage. Nursing Standard 5(44): 26–8.

Kohler-Ockmore J, Feneley RCL (1996) Long-term catheterisation of bladder: prevalence and morbidity. British Journal of Urology 77: 347–51.

Laker C (ed) (1994) Urological Nursing. London: Scutari Press.

Laurent C. (1998) (i) Preventing infection from indwelling catheters. (ii) Catheters: making the right choice. Nursing Times 94(25): 60–6.

Lavelle-Jones C, Byrne DJ, Rice P, Cushieri A (1993) Factors affecting the quality of informed consent. British Medical Journal 306: 885–90.

Leiter E, Futterwiet W, Brown GR (1993) Gender reassignment: psychiatric, endocrinologic and surgical management. Reconstructive Urology 2: 921–32.

Lepor H, Brewer MK, McConnel JD, Oesterling J (1992) What will replace TURP? Contemporary Urology 4(2): 30–40.

Lever R (1996) Cranberry juice. Professional Nurse 11(8): 525–6.

Lind J, Nakao SL (1990) Urologic and Male Genital Cancers, 2nd edn. Boston, MA: Jones and Bartlett.

Long B, Phipps W (1995) Adult Nursing: A Nursing Process Approach. London: Mosby.

Lowthian P (1998) The dangers of long-term catheter drainage. British Journal of Nursing 7(7): 366–79.

Lue T (1991) Physiology of penile erection. In Jonas U, Thon WF, Steif CG (eds) Erectile Dysfunction. Berlin: Springer-Verlag.

Luker K, Caress AL (1989) Rethinking patient education. Journal of Advanced Nursing 14: 711–18.

McCance KL, Huether S (1994) Pathophysiology: The Biologic Basis for Disease in Adults and Children. St Louis: Mosby.

MacKenzie J, Webb C (1995) Gynopia in nursing practice: the case of urethral catheterisation. Journal of Clinical Nursing 4: 221–6.

Maizels M, Reisman EM, Flom LS, Nelson J, Fernbach S, Firlit CF (1992) Grading nephroureteral dilatations detected in the first year of life – correlation with obstruction. Journal of Urology 148: 609.

Mansi MK, Alkhudair WK (1997) Conservative management with percutaneous intervention of major blunt renal injuries. American Journal of Emergency Medicine 15(7): 633–7.

May C (1995) Patient autonomy and the politics of professional relationships. Journal of Advanced Nursing 21: 83–7.

Mitchell ME, Close CE (1996) Early ablation for posterior urethral valves. Seminars in Pediatric Surgery 5(1): 66–71.

Molin C (1996) The special case of clinical trials. European Journal of Cancer Care 5(Suppl. 1): 1–8.

Morris N, Stickler D, Winters C (1997) Which indwelling urethral catheters resist encrustation by Proteus mirabilis biofilms? British Journal of Urology 80: 58–63.

Mouriquand PDE, Thomas DFM (1997) Posterior urethral valves and other congenital abnormalities of the urethra. In Thomas DFM (ed) Urological Disease in the Fetus and Infant Diagnosis and Management. Oxford: Butterworth-Heinemann.

Murphy K, Malloy T (1987) Bladder outlet obstruction. In Hanno PM, Wein AJ (eds) A Clinical Manual of Urology. Connecticut: Appleton Century Crofts.

Neal AJ, Hoskin PJ (1997) Clinical Oncology: Basic Principles and Practices. London: Arnold.

Nichols P (1988) Pathology of cancer of the penis. In Skinner DG, Lieskovsky G (eds) Diagnosis and Management of Genitourinary Cancer. Philadelphia, PA: WB Saunders.

Nielson B (1992) Applying andragogy in nursing continuing education. Journal of Continuing Education in Nursing 23(4): 148–51.

Ozdemir E (1997) Significantly increased complication risks with mass circumcision. British Journal of Urology 80: 136–9.

Pearson S, Goulart-Fisher D, Lee T (1995) Critical pathways as a strategy for improving care: problems and potential. Annals of Internal Medicine 123: 941–8.

Peate I (1997) Patient management following suprapubic catheterisation. British Journal of Nursing 6(10): 555–62.

Piemme JA (1988) Prostate cancer. In Baird SB (ed) Decision Making in Oncology Nursing. Toronto: BC Decker.

Pomfret I (1991) The catheter debate. Nursing Times 87(37): 67–8.

Porter S (1994) New nursing: the road to freedom? Journal of Advanced Nursing 20: 269–74.

Quaglia MP (1996) Genitourinary cancers in childhood. Seminars in Pediatric Surgery 5(1): 49–65.

Ragozzino D, Testa G, de-Ritis R et al. (1997) Severe obliteration of the urethral lumen after wall stent insertion. Aktuelle Radiol 7(4): 179–82.

Rankin SH, Duffy KL (1983) Patient Education Issues, Principles and Guidelines. Philadelphia: JB Lippincott.

Ransley PG, Duffy PG, Wollin M (1989) Bladder exstrophy closure and epispadias repair. In Spitz L (ed) Operative Surgery – Pediatric Surgery, pp 627–32. London: Butterworth.

Ream E, Richardson A (1996) The role of information in patients' adaptation to chemotherapy and radiotherapy: a review of the literature. European Journal of Cancer Care 5: 132–8.

Redman B (1993) Patient education at 25 years; where we have been and where we are going. Journal of Advanced Nursing 18: 725–30.

Reilly NJ (1995) Genitourinary trauma. In Karlowicz KA (ed) Urologic Nursing: Principles and Practice. London: WB Saunders.

Rickwood AMK (1989) Circumcision of boys in England: current practice. Pediatric Surgery International 4: 231–2.

Rickwood AMK (1992) The unkindest cut of all. Journal of the Irish College of Physicians and Surgeons 21(3): 179–80.

Rickwood AMK (1997) Congenital disorders of the bladder. In Thomas DFM (ed) Urological Disease in the Fetus and Infant Diagnosis and Management. Oxford: Butterworth-Heinemann.

Rickwood AMK, Godiwalla SY (1998) The natural history of pelvic–ureteric junction obstruction in children presenting clinically with the complaint. British Journal of Urology 80: 793–6.

Rigby D (1998) Long-term catheter care. Professional Nurse 13(5): S14–S15.

Rodwell C (1996) An analysis of the concept of empowerment. Journal of Advanced Nursing 23: 305–13.

Roe B, Reid F, Brocklehurst J (1988) Comparison of four urine drainage systems. Journal of Advanced Nursing 13: 374–82.

Rogers A (1993) Legal implications of transsexualism. Lancet 341: 1085–6.

Roper N, Logan W, Tierney A (1990) The Elements of Nursing, 3rd edn. Edinburgh: Churchill Livingstone.

Rose P (1992) Care of a child with hypospadias: ethical issues in practice. British Journal of Nursing 1(8): 393–8.

Rosella JD (1994) Testicular cancer health education: an integrative review. Journal of Advanced Nursing 20: 666–71.

Rosenberg SA, Lotze MT, Yang JC (1989) Combination therapy with interleukin-2 and alpha-interferon for the treatment of patients with advanced cancer. Journal of Clinical Oncology 7: 1863–74.

Royal College of Nursing (1997) Continence Care Forum. Male Catheterisation, the Role of the Nurse. London: RCN.

Safak T, Yuksel E, Ozcan G, Gursu G (1996) Utilization of the breast for penile reconstruction in a transsexual. Plastic and Reconstructive Surgery 96(6): 1483–5.

Sagalowsky AL, Milam H, Reveley R, Silva FG (1982) Prediction of lymphatic metastases by the Gleason histological grading in prostatic cancer. Journal of Urology 128: 951–2.

Schellhammer PF et al. (1992) Tumours of the Penis: Campbell's Urology. Philadelphia, PA: WB Saunders.

Simpson PE (ed) (1998) Introduction to Surgical Nursing. London: Arnold.

Slag MF, Morley JE, Elson MK et al. (1983) Impotence in medical clinic outpatients. Journal of the American Medical Association 249: 1736–40.

Smith C (1989) Overview of patient education. Nursing Clinics of North America 24(3): 583–7.

Squire R (1997) Genitourinary malignancies in the first year of life. In Thomas DFM (ed) Urological Disease in the Fetus and Infant Diagnosis and Management. Oxford: Butterworth-Heinemann.

Steggall M (1999) TUR syndrome: a risk after prostatic surgery. Professional Nurse 14(5): 323–6.

Taylor TK (1991) Endocrine therapy for advanced stage D prostate cancer. Urological Nursing 11(3): 22–6.

Teasdale K (1993) Information and anxiety: a critical reappraisal. Journal of Advanced Nursing 18: 1125–32.

Thomas DFM (1997) Vesicoureteric reflux. In Thomas DFM (ed) Urological Disease in the Fetus and Infant Diagnosis and Management. Oxford: Butterworth-Heinemann.

Thomas DFM, Barker AP (1997) Incidence: facts and figures. In Thomas DFM (ed) Urological Disease in the Fetus and Infant Diagnosis and Management. Oxford: Butterworth-Heinemann.

Tilley JD, Gregor FM, Thiessen V (1987) The nurse's role in patient education: incongruent perceptions amongst nurses and patients. Journal of Advanced Nursing 12: 291–301.

UKCC (1992) The Scope of Professional Practice. London: UKCC.

UKCC (1996) Guidelines for Professional Practice. London: UKCC.

USDOH (1991) Urinary Tract Infection in Adults. United States Department of Health and Human Services Publications.

Uygur MC, Gulerkaya B, Altag U et al. (1997) 13 years experience of penile fracture. Scandinavian Journal of Urology and Nephrology 31(3): 265–6.

Vaughn ED (eds) Campbell's Urology, 6th edn. Philadelphia, PA: WB Saunders.

Waller L, Telander M, Sullivan L (1997) The importance of osmolality in hydrophilic catheters: a cross over study. Spinal Cord 35(4): 229–33.

Walsh PC (1986) Radical retropubic prostatectomy. In Walsh PC, Retik AB, Stamey TA.

Walters WAW, Ross MW (1986) Transsexualism and Sex Reassignment. Oxford: Oxford University Press.

Watson JE (1979) Medical Surgical Nursing and Related Physiology, 2nd edn. Philadelphia, PA: WB Saunders.

Whitaker RH, Williams DM (1997) Postnatal investigation and management of genital and intersex anomalies. In Thomas DFM (ed) Urological Disease in the Fetus and Infant Diagnosis and Management. Oxford: Butterworth-Heinemann.

Wigfield A, Boon E (1996) Critical care pathway development: the way forward. British Journal of Nursing 15(12): 732–5.

Wilde M (1997) Long-term indwelling urinary catheter care: conceptualising the research base. Journal of Advanced Nursing 25: 1252–61.

Willard C (1995) Informed consent in the oncology setting. Journal of Cancer Care 4: 147–51.

Willis J (1995a) Catheters: product selection. Nursing Times 91(9): 45–6.

Willis J (1995b) Catheters: urinary tract infections. Nursing Times 91(35): 48–9.

Willis J (1996) Continence: intermittent self catheterisation. Nursing Times 92(33): 56–8.

Willis J (1998) Promoting continence control. Nursing Times 94(15): 59–60.

Wilson-Barnett J (1985) Principles of patient teaching. Nursing Times 81: 28–9.

Winder A (1994) An unsuitable job for a woman? Nursing Times 90(22): 46–8.

Winn C (1996) Basing catheter care on research principles. Nursing Standard 10(18): 38–40.

Winn C (1998) Complications with urinary catheters. Professional Nurse 13(5): S7–S10.

Winn C, Thompson J (1998) Urinary catheter for intermittent use. Professional Nurse 13(8): 541–8.

Winson L (1997) Catheterisation: a need for improved patient management. British Journal of Nursing 6(21): 1225–52.

Woodhouse CRJ (1989) Sexual rehabilitation in bladder exstrophy. In Eicher W (ed) Plastic Surgery in the Sexually Handicapped. Berlin: Springer-Verlag.

Woodward S (1997) Complications of allergies to latex urinary catheters. British Journal of Nursing 6(14): 786–92.

Woollons S (1996) Urinary catheters for long-term use. Professional Nurse 11(12): 825–32.

Glossary of terms

Abdomen The area between the diaphragm and the pelvis.

Abscess A localized collection of pus.

Acid A proton donor, or substance that dissociates into hydrogen ions (H^+) and anions (negatively charged ions); characterized by an excess of hydrogen ions and a pH less than 7.

Adrenal glands Two glands located superior to each kidney. Also called the suprarenal glands.

Adrenaline Neurotransmitter and hormone; released from the neurons of the sympathetic nervous system and from the adrenal medulla. Also called epinephrine.

Afferent arteriole A blood vessel of the kidney that breaks up into a capillary network called a glomerulus; there is one afferent arteriole for each glomerulus.

Aldosterone A mineralocorticoid produced by the adrenal cortex that brings about sodium and water reabsorption and potassium excretion.

Alimentary Pertaining to nutrition.

Angioplasty Surgery of blood vessels, aimed at widening the lumen.

Angiotensin Either of two forms of a protein associated with regulation of blood pressure. Angiotensin I is produced by the action of renin on angiotensinogen and is converted by the action of a plasma enzyme into angiotensin II, which stimulates aldosterone secretion by the adrenal cortex.

Anterior Nearer to or at the front of the body. Also called ventral.

Antidiuretic hormone (ADH) Hormone produced by neurosecretory cells in the paraventricular and supraoptic nuclei of the hypothalmus that stimulates water reabsorption from kidney cells into the blood and vasoconstriction of arterioles.

Aorta The main systemic trunk of the arteriole system of the body that emerges from the left ventricle.

Artery A blood vessel that carries blood away from the heart.

Atrophy A wasting or a reduction in an organ or tissue.

Azoospermia Non-production of spermatozoa.

Balanitis xerosis obliterans A non-infective, aggressive fibrosis of the foreskin.

Bladder diverticulum Herniation of the mucosa of the bladder wall.

Bladder exstrophy A failure or incomplete closure of the lower anterior abdominal wall.

Bowman's capsule A double-walled globe at the proximal end of a nephron that encloses the glomerulus.

Calcitonin A hormone produced by the thyroid gland that lowers the calcium and phosphate levels of the blood by inhibiting bone breakdown and accelerating calcium absorption by bones.

Clitoris An erectile organ of the female, located at the anterior junction of the labia minora that is homologous to the male penis.

Cortex An outer layer of an organ. The convoluted layer of grey matter covering each cerebral hemisphere.

Counter current mechanism One mechanism involved in the ability of the kidneys to produce a hyperosmotic urine.

Cryptorchidism Undescended testes.

Cystitis Inflammation of the bladder.

Cystogram X-ray test involving the instillation of a radio-opaque dye into the bladder.

Cystotomy Surgical opening of the bladder.

Diaphragm Any partition that separates one area from another, especially the dome-shaped skeletal muscle between the thoracic and abdominal cavities. Also a dome-shaped structure that fits over the cervix, usually with a spermicide, to prevent conception.

Diffusion Movement of molecules down a concentration gradient from a higher concentration to a lower concentration until equilibrium is achieved.

Diverticulum A pouch or pocket in the lining of a hollow organ.

Duodenum The first 25 cm (10 in) of the small intestine.

Dysfunction Impairment of function.

Efferent arteriole A vessel of the renal vascular system that transports blood from the glomerulus to the peritubular capillary.

Electrolyte Any compound that separates into ions when dissolved in water and is able to conduct electricity.

Enterocystoplasty Reconstruction of the bladder using bowel.

Epididymis A comma-shaped organ that lies along the posterior border of the testis and contains the ductus epididymis, in which the sperm undergo maturation. Plural, epididymides.

Epispadias The penile urethra opens on the dorsal penis.

External Located on or near the surface.

Faeces Waste material discharged from the large intestine; excrement; stool.

Fascia A fibrous membrane covering, supporting, and separating muscles.

Feedback system A sequence of events in which information about the status of a situation is continually reported (fed back) to a central control region.

Glans penis The slightly enlarged region at the distal end of the penis.

Gleason score An indicator of prognosis.

Glomerular filtration The first step in urine formation in which substances in blood are filtered at the endothelial-capsular membrane and the filtrate enters the proximal convoluted tubule of a nephron.

Glucocorticoids Hormones secreted by the cortex of the adrenal gland, especially cortisol, that influence glucose metabolism.

Gynaecomastia True, palpable and sometimes tender breast tissue in a male.

Haematogenous Originating from the blood.

Haematuria Blood in the urine.

Heart A hollow muscular organ lying slightly to the left of the midline of the chest that pumps the blood through the cardiovascular system.

Hepatomegaly Liver enlargement.

Hirsutism Excessive hairiness, especially in women.

Histology The study of cell structure.

Hydrocele Fluid accumulation between the layers of the tunica vaginalis.

Hydrocelectomy Removal of the accumulated fluid between the layers of the tunica vaginalis.

Hydronephrosis Swelling and enlargement of the kidney due to formed urine being unable to leave and back pressure developing.

Hyperplasia Excessive formation of normal cells which leads to increase in size.

Hypogonadism A hypothalamic-pituitary disorder.

Hypospadias The penile urethra opens ventrally anywhere between the glans and perineum.

Ileal conduit Stoma created for the continuous drainage of urine.

Infarction An area of necrotic tissue due to occlusion.

Inferior Away from the head or towards the lower part of a structure. Also called caudal.

Inferior vena cava (IVC) Large vein that collects blood from parts of the body inferior to the heart and returns it to the right atrium.

Inguinal canal An oblique passageway in the anterior abdominal wall just superior and parallel to the medial half of the inguinal ligament that transmits the spermatic cord and ilioinguinal nerve in the male and round ligament of the uterus and ilioinguinal nerve in the female.

Internal Away from the surface of the body.

Intravesical Into the bladder.

Ischaemia A deficiency in or lack of blood supply to a part of the body.

Jejunum The middle portion of the small intestine.

Juxtaglomerular apparatus (JGA) Consists of the macula densa (cells of the distal convoluted tubule adjacent to the afferent and efferent arterioles) and juxtaglomerular cells (modified cells of the afferent and sometimes efferent arteriole); secretes renin when blood pressure starts to fall.

Kidney One of the paired reddish coloured organs located in the lumbar region that regulate the composition and volume of blood and produce urine.

Litholapaxy Crushing of a bladder stone in theatre.

Liver Large gland under the diaphragm, which occupies most of the right hypochondriac region and part of the epigastric region. Functionally, it produces bile salts, heparin and plasma proteins; converts one nutrient into another; detoxifies substances; stores glycogen, minerals and vitamins; carries on phagocytosis of blood cells and bacteria; and helps activate vitamin D.

Malignancy A virulent growth of cells, i.e. a cancer.

Mammoplasty Construction of breasts.

Medulla An inner layer of an organ, such as the medulla of the kidney.

Metastases Secondary deposits of tumours that occur away from the primary tumour.

Micturition The act of expelling urine from the urinary bladder. Also called urination.

Mineralocorticoids A group of hormones of the adrenal cortex.

Mitrofanoff stoma A continent diversion for urinary output.

Necrosis Death of tissue.

Nephrectomy Removal of the kidney.

Nephrolithiasis Stone in the kidney(s).

Nephron The functional unit of the kidney.

Nesbit's plication Operation to correct the curvature caused by Peyronies disease.

Norepinephrine (NE) A hormone secreted by the adrenal medulla that produces actions similar to those that result from sympathetic stimulation. Also called noradrenaline.

Oophorectomy Removal of the ovaries.

Orchidectomy Surgical removal of one or both testicles.

Orchidopexy Fixation of one or both of the testicles in the scrotum.

Orchitis Inflammation of the testis.

Orifice Any aperture or opening.

Osmosis Movement of water molecules across a selectively permeable membrane from an area of high concentration of water molecules (a dilute solution) to an area of low concentration of water molecules (a concentrated solution).

Osteomalacia Painful softening of bones due to vitamin D deficiency.

Pancreas A soft oblong organ lying along the greater curvature of the stomach and connected by a duct to the duodenum. It is both exocrine (secreting pancreatic juice) and endocrine (secreting insulin, glucagon, growth hormone inhibiting hormone and pancreatic polypeptide).

Paraphimosis The inability to replace the foreskin in its normal position.

Parietal Pertaining to or forming the outer wall of a body cavity.

Penectomy Amputation of the penis.

Penis The male copulatory organ, used to introduce spermatozoa into the female vagina.

Peritoneum The largest serous membrane of the body. It lines the abdominal cavity and covers the viscera.

Peyronies disease Curvature of the erect penis.

Phimosis Inability to retract the foreskin.

Posterior Nearer to or at the back of the body. Also called dorsal.

Priapism Persistent erection of the penis (usually without sexual desire).

Prostate gland A doughnut-shaped gland inferior to the urinary bladder that surrounds the superior portion of the male urethra and secretes a slightly acid solution that contributes to sperm motility and viability.

Prostatic hyperplasia Enlargement of the prostate gland.

Prostatitis Inflammation of the prostate.

Prostatodynia Painful prostate.

Prosthesis An artificial part fitted to the body.

Prune-belly syndrome Deficient abdominal wall musculature.

Pyelonephritis Infection and inflamation of the kidney and renal pelvis.

Rectum The last 20 cm (7 in) of the gastrointestinal tract, from the sigmoid colon to the anus.

Renal Pertaining to the kidney.

Renal pelvis A cavity in the centre of the kidney formed by the expanded, proximal portion of the ureter, lying within the kidney, and into which the major calyces open.

Renal pyramid A triangular structure in the renal medulla composed of the straight segments of the renal tubules.

Renin An enzyme released by the kidney into the plasma, where it converts angiotensinogen into angiotensin I.

Retrograde ejaculation Expulsion of semen into the bladder as opposed to via the urethral opening.

Retroperitoneal fibrosis Formation of fibrous tissue behind the peritoneum, which can lead to compression and distortion of the ureters.

Salpingectomy Removal of the Fallopian tubes.

Scrotum A skin-covered pouch that contains the testes and their accessory structures.

Secretion Production and release of a fluid from a gland, especially a functionally useful product as opposed to a waste product.

Seminal vesicle One of a pair of convoluted, pouch-like structures, lying posterior and inferior to the urinary bladder and anterior to the rectum, that secrete a component of semen into the ejaculatory ducts.

Sertoli cells Non-dividing support cells, enabling development of spermatids into sperm within the seminiferous tubules.

Sinus A hollow in a bone (paranasal sinus) or other tissue; a channel for blood (vascular sinus); any cavity having a narrow opening.

Spermatic cord A supporting structure of the male reproductive system, extending from the testes to the deep inguinal ring, that includes the ductus (vas) deferens, arteries, veins, lymphatic vessels, nerves, cremaster muscle and connective tissue.

Spermatids Secondary spermatocytes having undergone meiosis.

Spermatocytes Large cells arising from spermatagonium.

Spermatogenesis Production of spermatozoa within the seminiferous tubules of the testis.

Spermatogonium Sperm cells nearest to the walls of the seminiferous tubules.

Spermatozoon A mature sperm cell. Plural, spermatozoa.

Spleen Large mass of lymphatic tissue between the fundus of the stomach and the diaphragm that functions in phagocytosis, production of lymphocytes and blood storage.

Superior Towards the head or upper part of the structure.

Suppuration The formation of pus.

T3 Transwave thermotherapy.

Tamponade The build up of fluid within a potential space, leading to pressure on adjacent organs/tissues.

Testosterone A male sex hormone (androgen) secreted by interstitial endocrinocytes (cells of Leydig) of a mature testis; controls the growth and development of male sex organs, secondary sex characteristics, spermatozoa and body growth.

Thermotherapy Heat treatment.

Transport maximum (TM) The maximum amount of a substance that can be reabsorbed by renal tubules under any condition.

Transsexualism The changing from one sex to the other.

Trigone A triangular area at the base of the urinary bladder.

Ureter One of two tubes that connect the kidney with the urinary bladder.

Ureterocele Cystic dilatation of the distal ureter.

Ureterolithiasis Stone in the ureter(s).

Uretero-ureterostomy Anastomosis of one ureter to the other.

Urethra The duct from the urinary bladder to the exterior of the body that conveys urine in females and urine and semen in males.

Urethrogram Examination of the urethra using a radio-opaque dye.

Urethroplasty Reconstruction of the urethra.

Urinary bladder A hollow, muscular organ situated in the pelvic cavity posterior to the pubic symphysis.

Urodynamics The study of bladder function.

Urolithiasis Stone in the urinary tract.

Vagina A muscular, tubular organ that leads from the uterus to the vestibule, situated between the urinary bladder and the rectum of the female.

Vaginectomy Removal of the vagina.

Varicocele A distension of the network of veins that form the venous network of the testes.

Vasectomy Surgical excision of a section of the vas deferens.

Vasovasostomy Surgical reversal of a vasectomy.

Vein A blood vessel that conveys blood from tissues back to the heart.

Vertebral column The 26 vertebrae; encloses and protects the spinal cord and serves as a point of attachment for the ribs and back muscles. Also called the spine, spinal column or backbone.

Voiding The act of expelling urine from the urinary bladder.

Index